Getting on wi[...]

Sheila Hollins, Jane Bernal, and
Alice Thacker,
illustrated by Lisa Kopper

Books Beyond Words

Gaskell/St George's Hospital Medical School
LONDON

First published in Great Britain 1999 by St George's Hospital Medical School and Gaskell.
Text & illustrations © Sheila Hollins 1999.

No part of this book may be reproduced in any form, or by any means without the prior permission in writing from the publisher.

Gaskell is a registered trademark of the Royal College of Psychiatrists.

The Royal College of Psychiatrists (no. 228636) and St George's Hospital Special Trustees (no. 241527) are registered charities.

British Library Cataloguing-in-Publication Data.
A catalogue record for this book is available from the British Library.
ISBN 1-901242-39-0

Distributed in North America
by American Psychiatric Press, Inc.

Printed and bound in Great Britain by Bell & Bain Limited, Thornliebank, Glasgow G46 7UQ.

Further information about the Books Beyond Words series can be obtained from:
Royal College of Psychiatrists
17 Belgrave Square
London SW1X 8PG
Tel: 0171 235 2351
Fax: 0171 245 1231

Acknowledgements

We would like to thank our editorial advisers, Peter McHugh, Eileen Smith, Nigel Hollins, Lloyd Page, Wendy Perez and the Women's Group and staff at Blakes & Link Employment Agency (Hammersmith & Fulham Social Services).

We are very grateful for the advice and support given to us by Dr Gus Baker, Dr Stephen Brown, Rebecca Chipere, Jane Edmonds, Leanda Evans, Catherine Gregory, Dr Yvonne Hart, Peter Holmes, and Dr Ekkehart Staufenberg.

Many people with epilepsy and learning disabilities helped us by trying out the illustrations while this book was in preparation. Their comments proved to be invaluable.

Our thanks also go to the staff in the MRI Departments of Atkinson Morleys Hospital and the National Hospital for Neurology and Neurosurgery.

Finally, we are grateful to Janssen-Cilag without whose generous financial support this book would not have been possible.

1

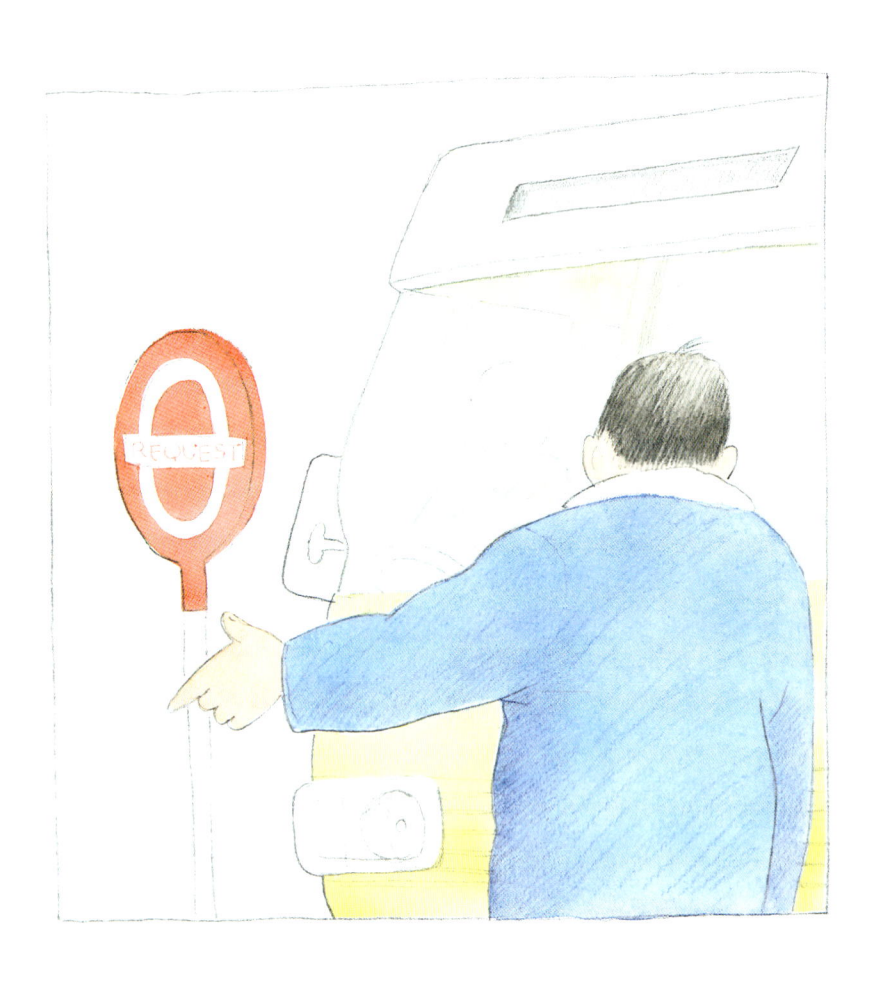

2

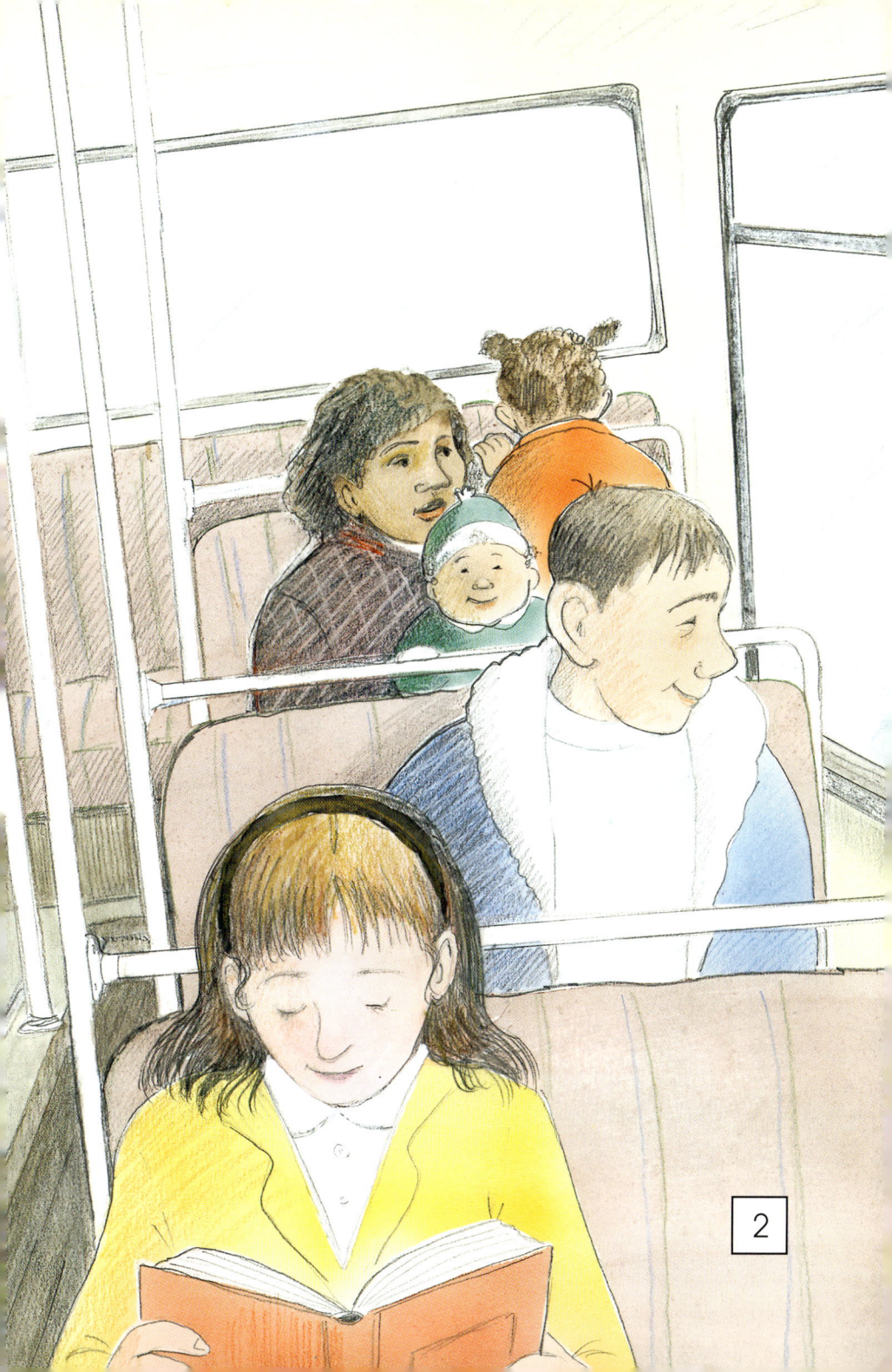

3

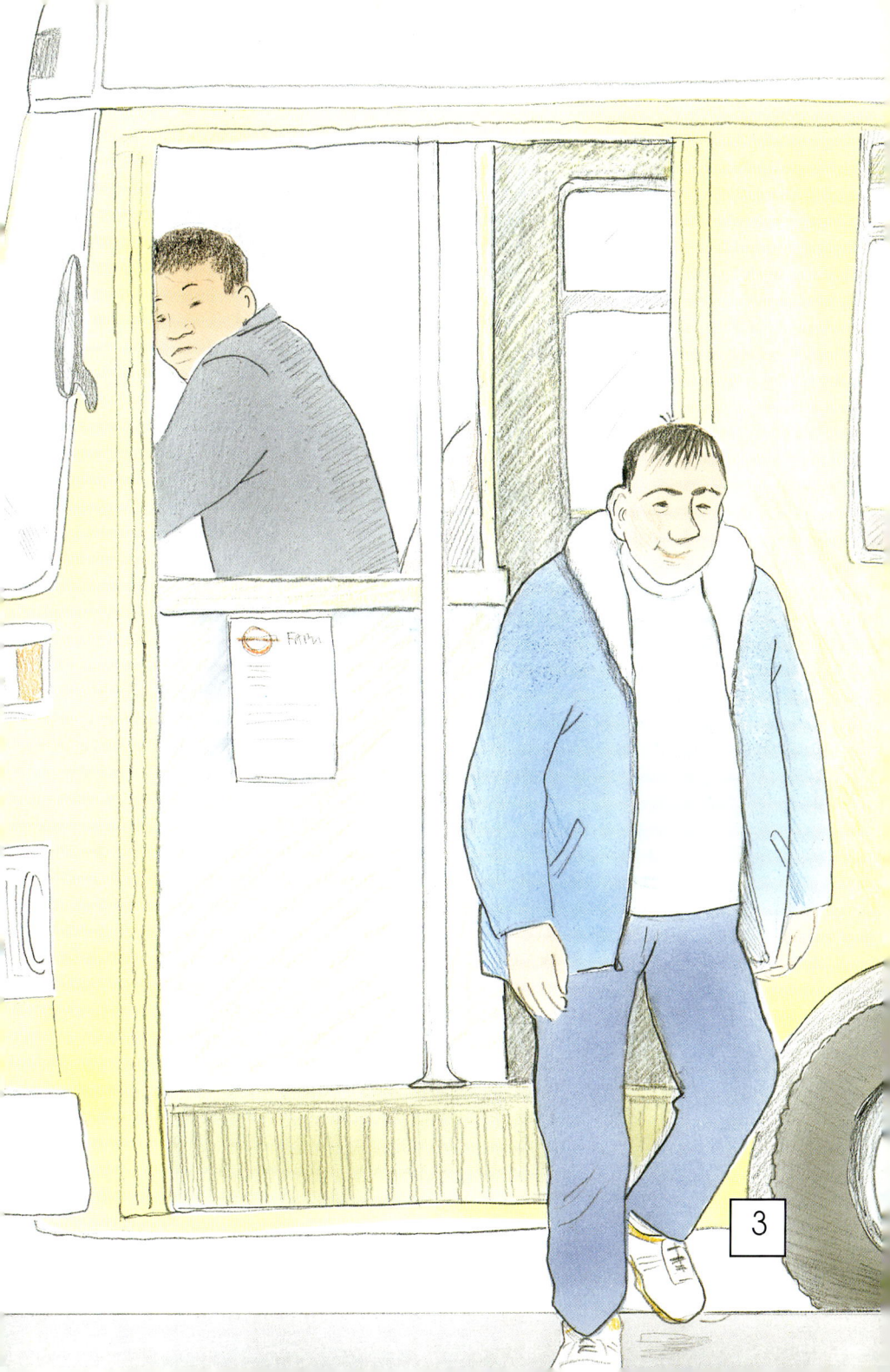

4

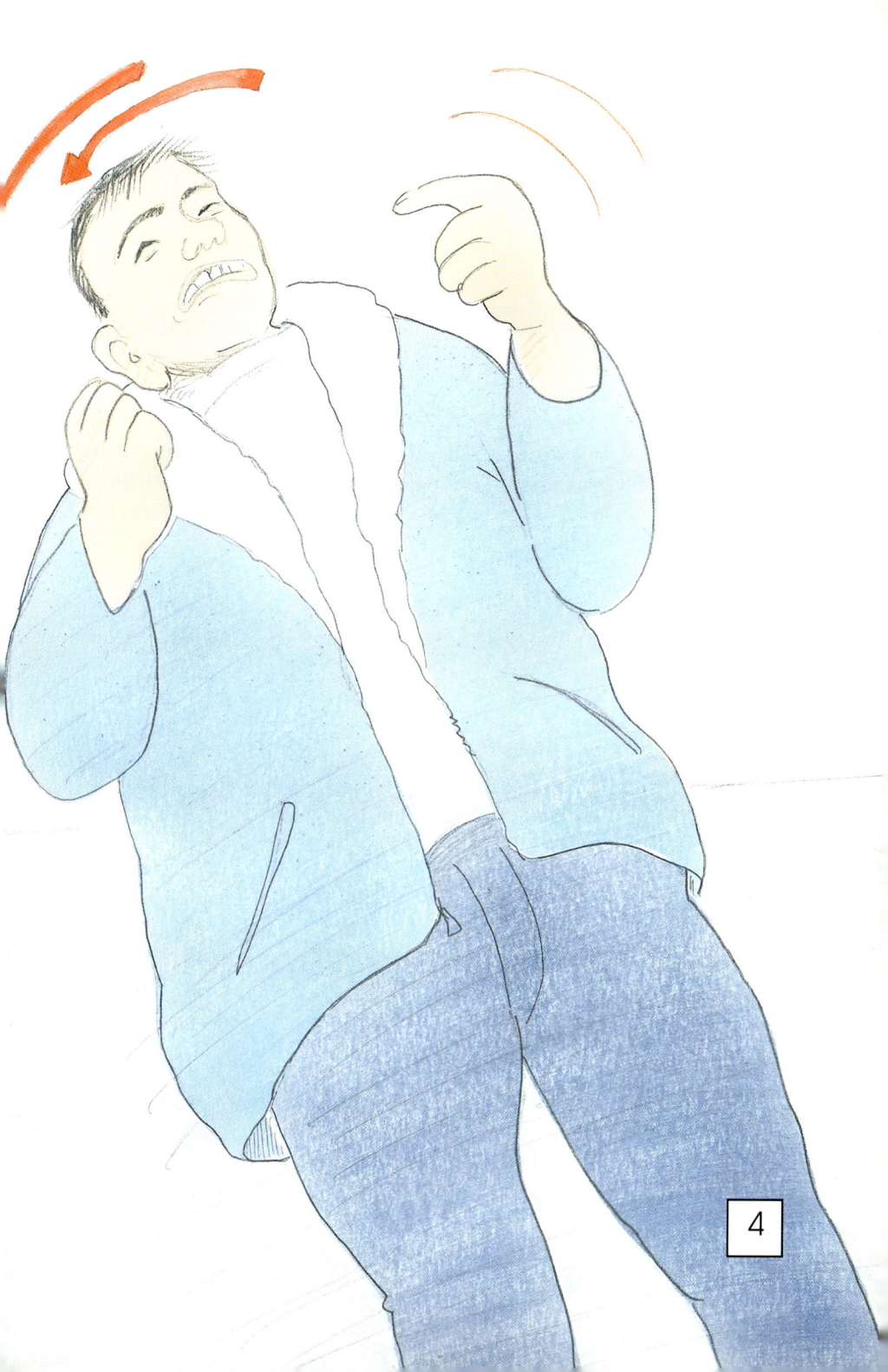

5

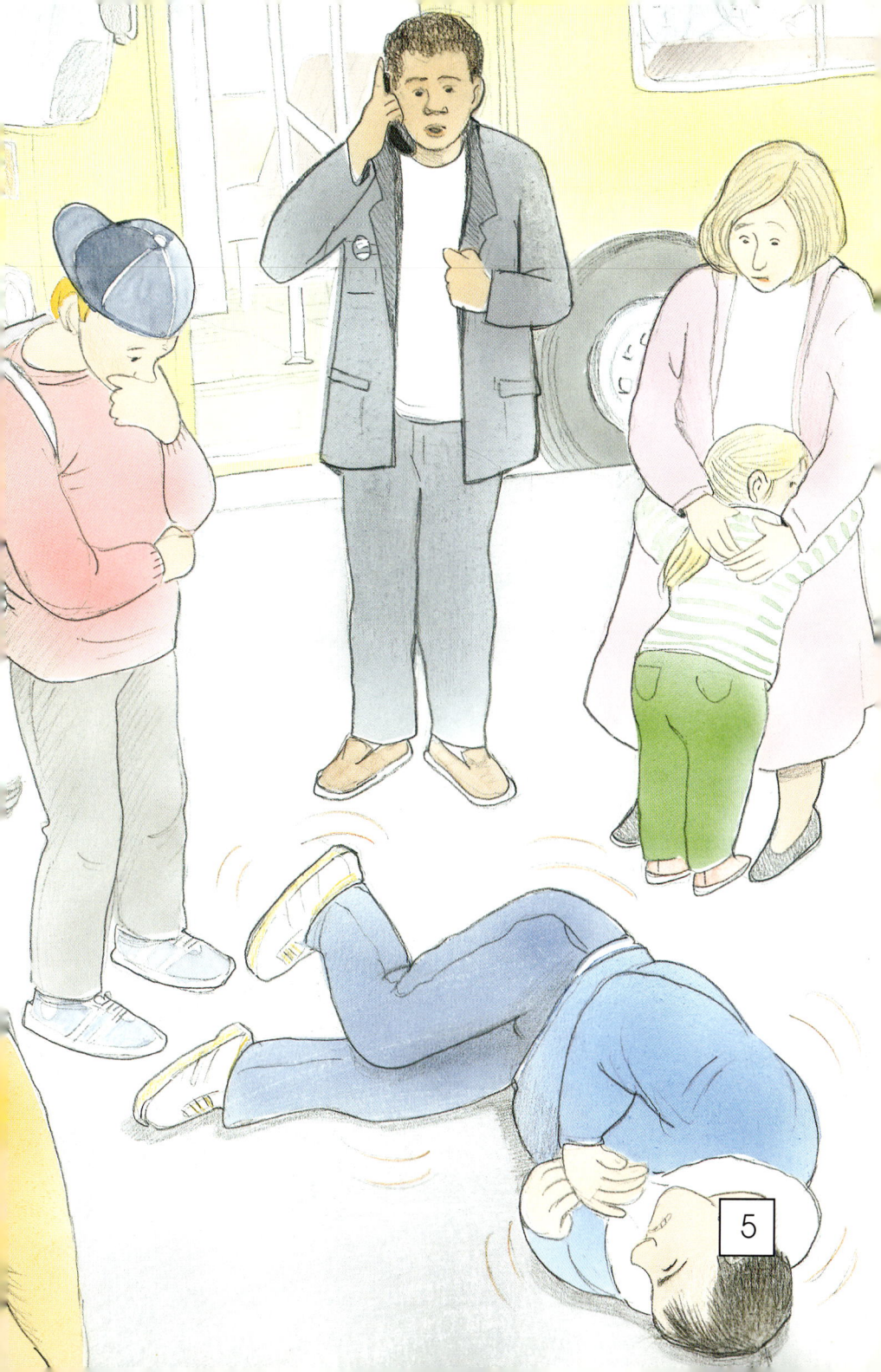

6

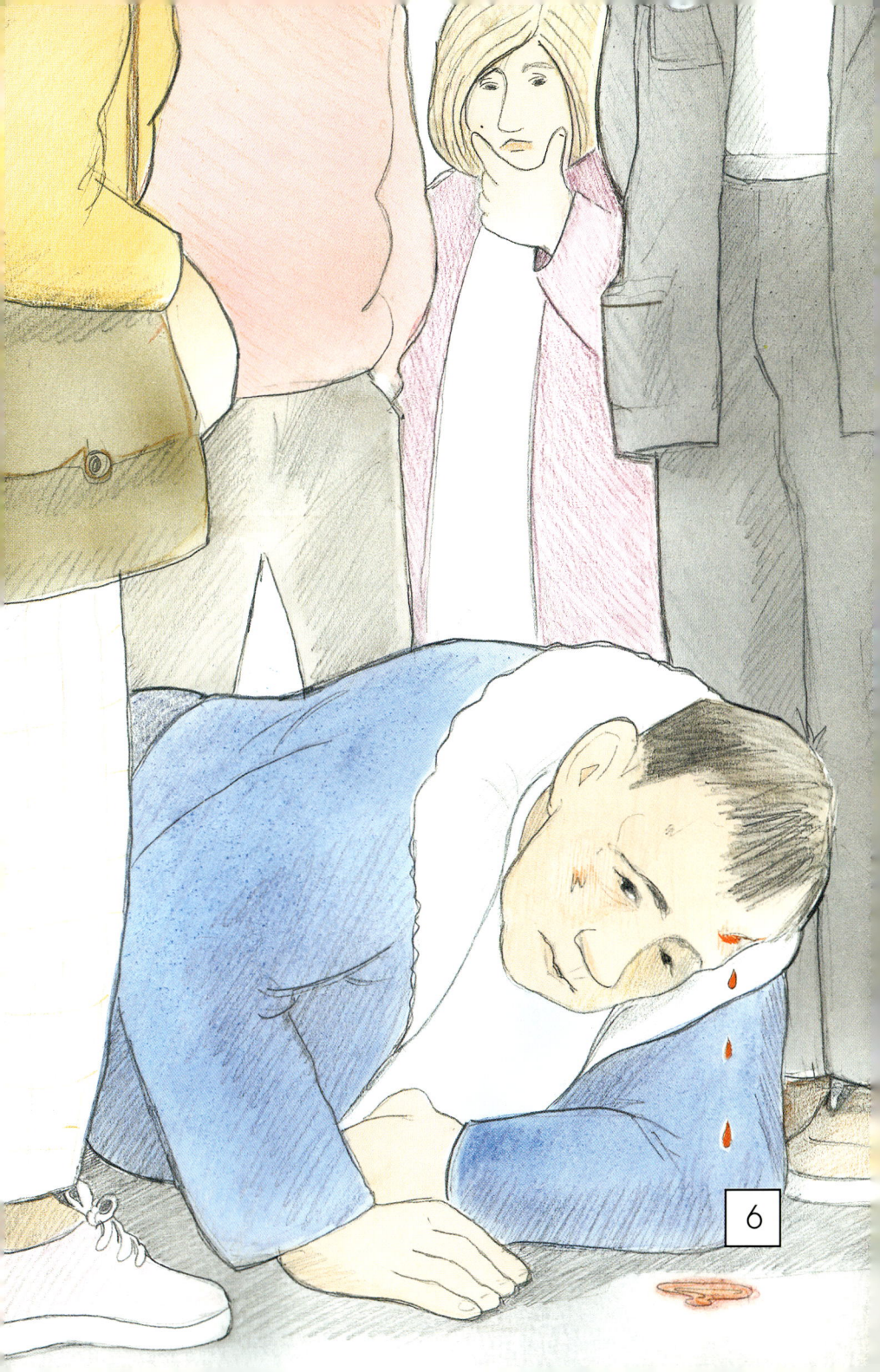

7

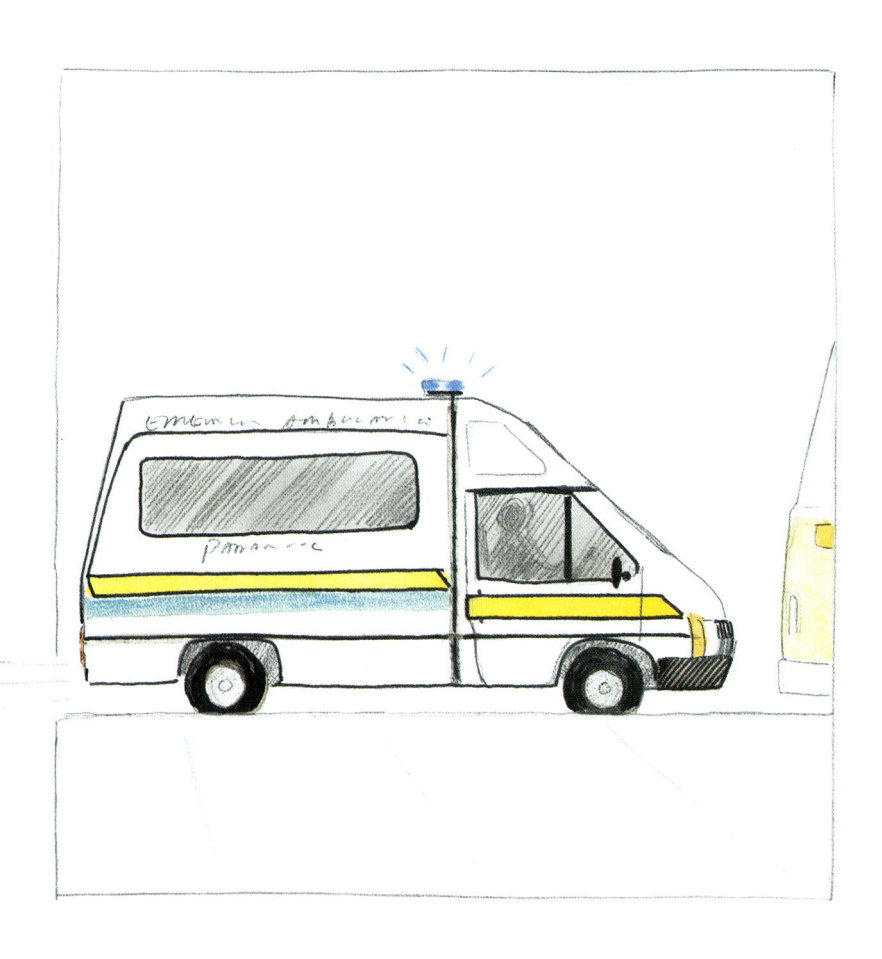

8

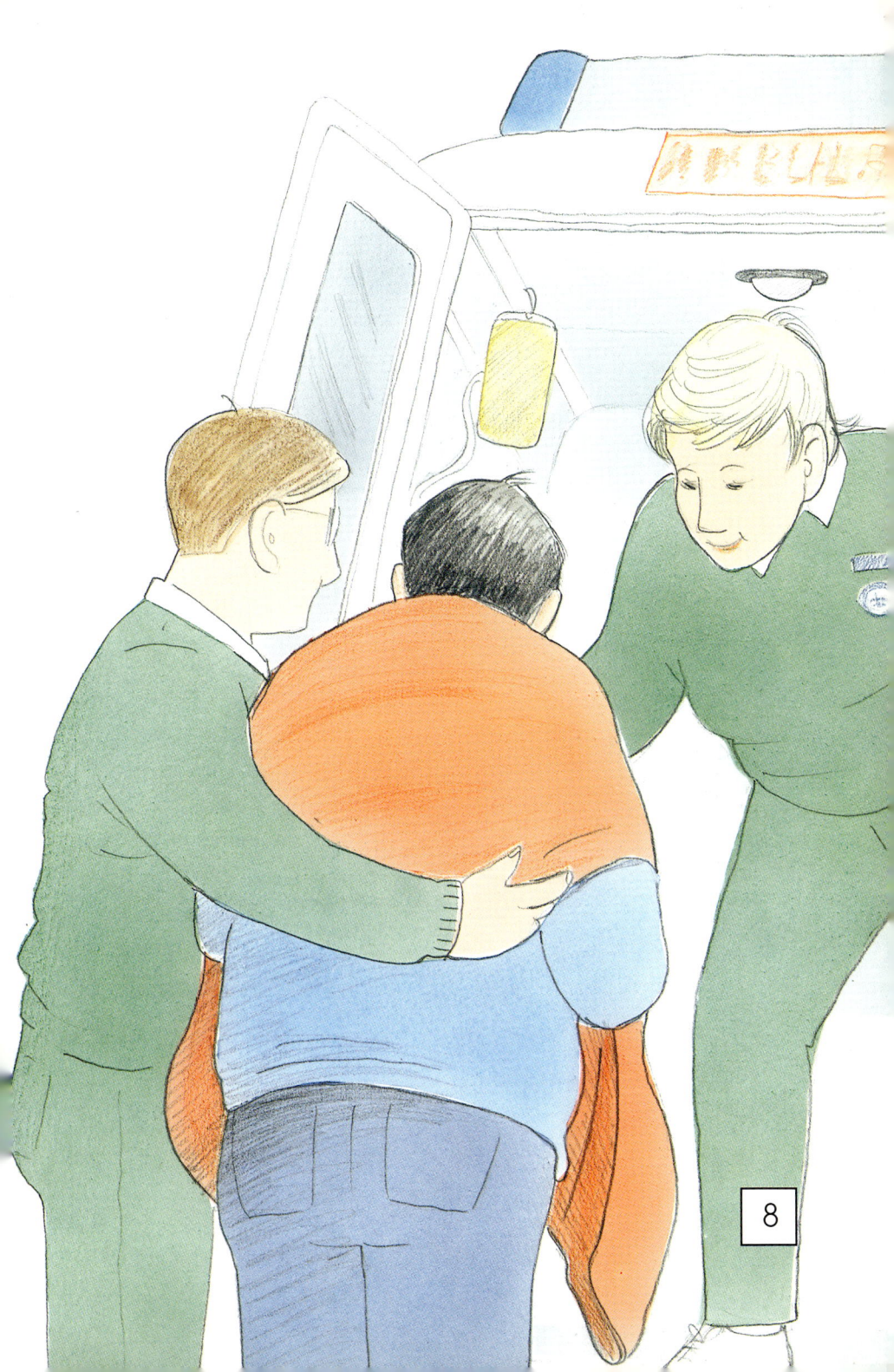

9

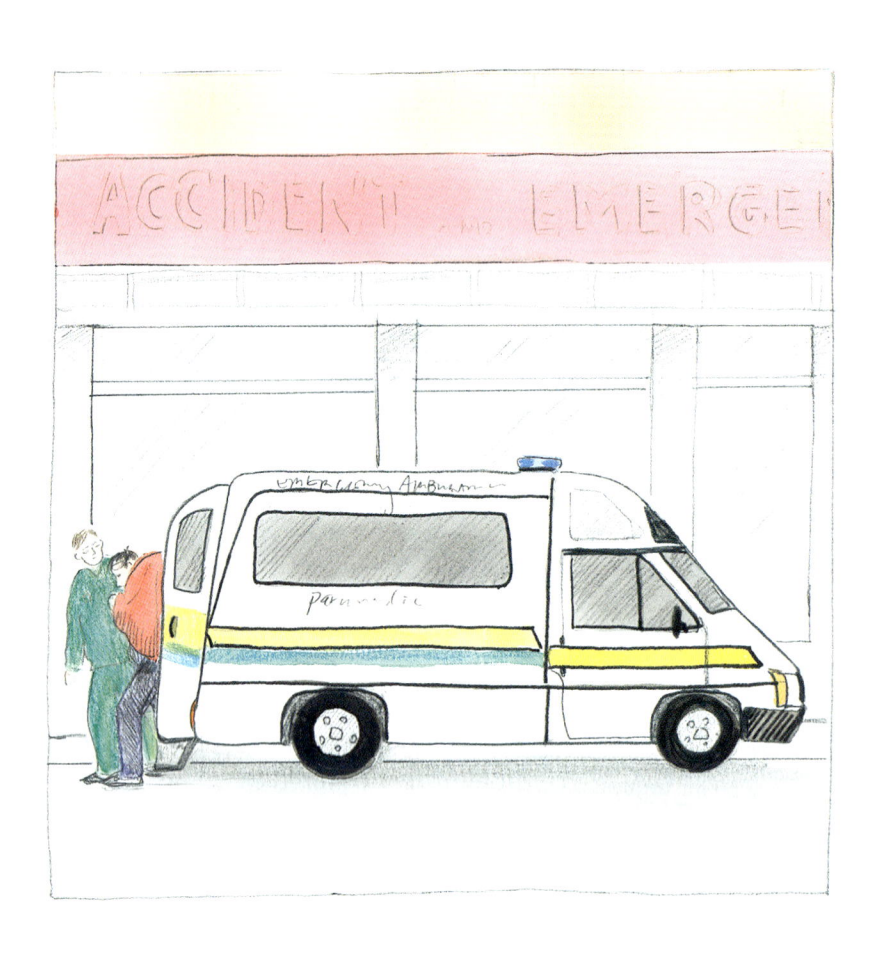

10

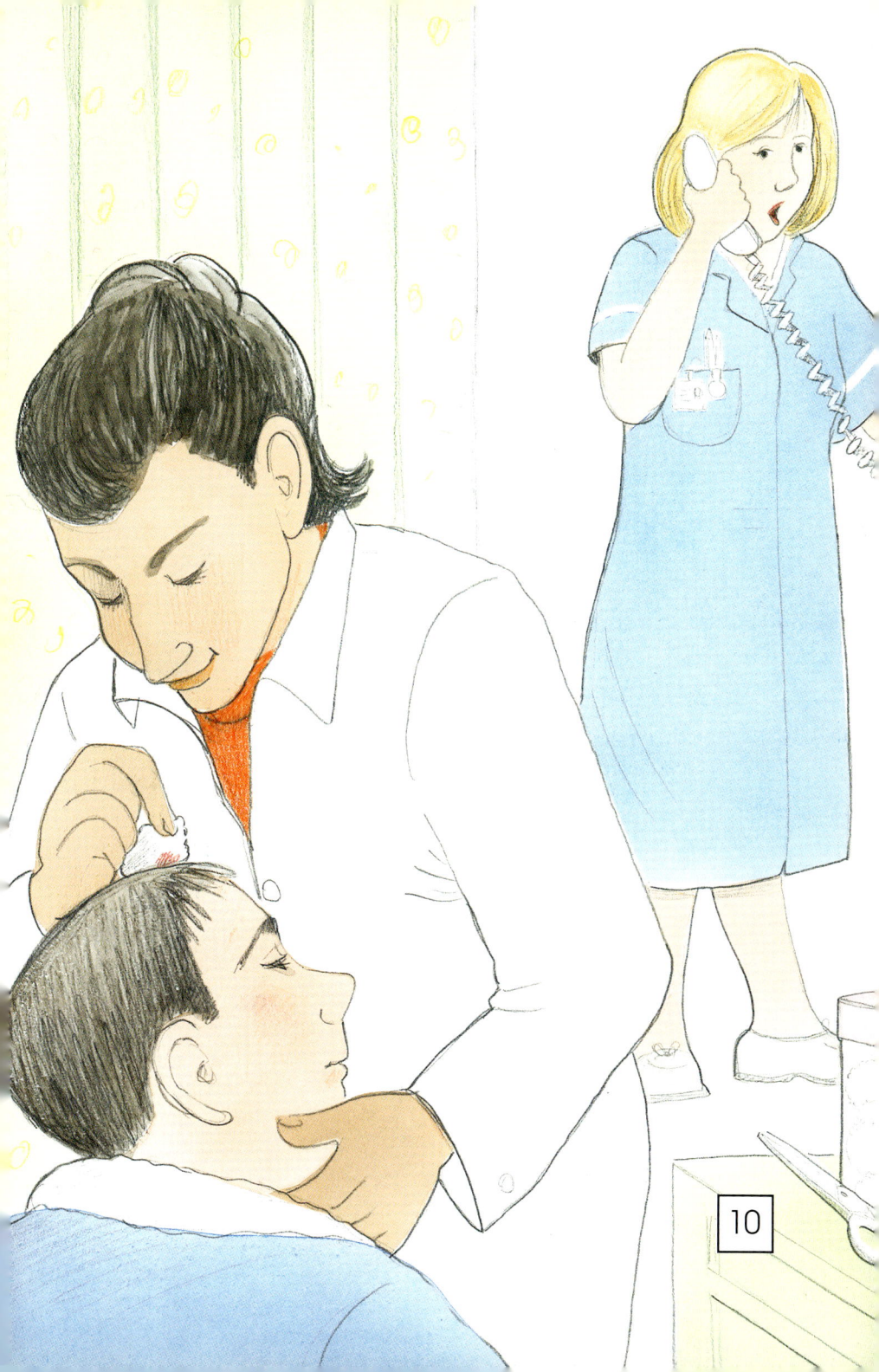

11

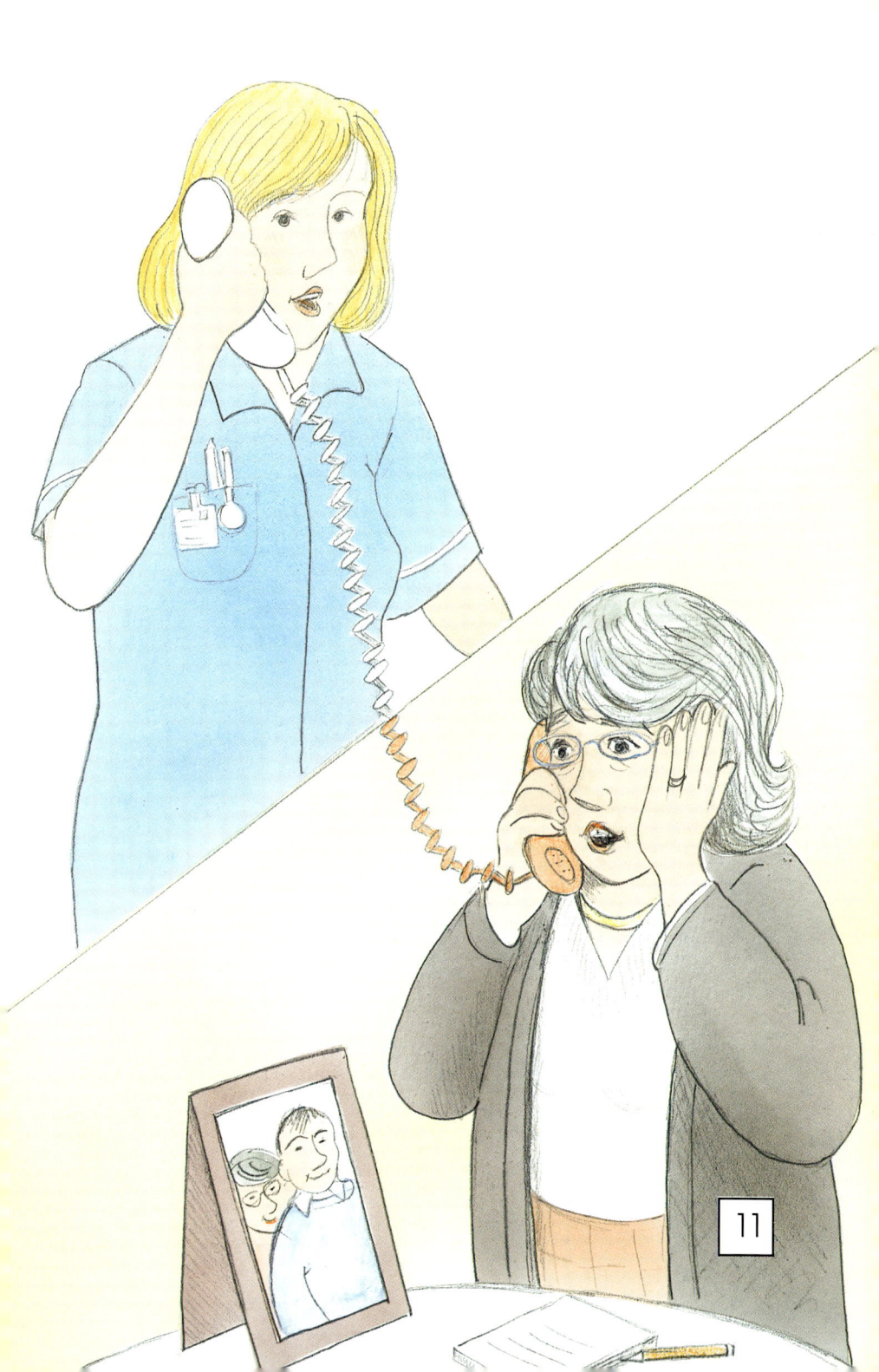

12

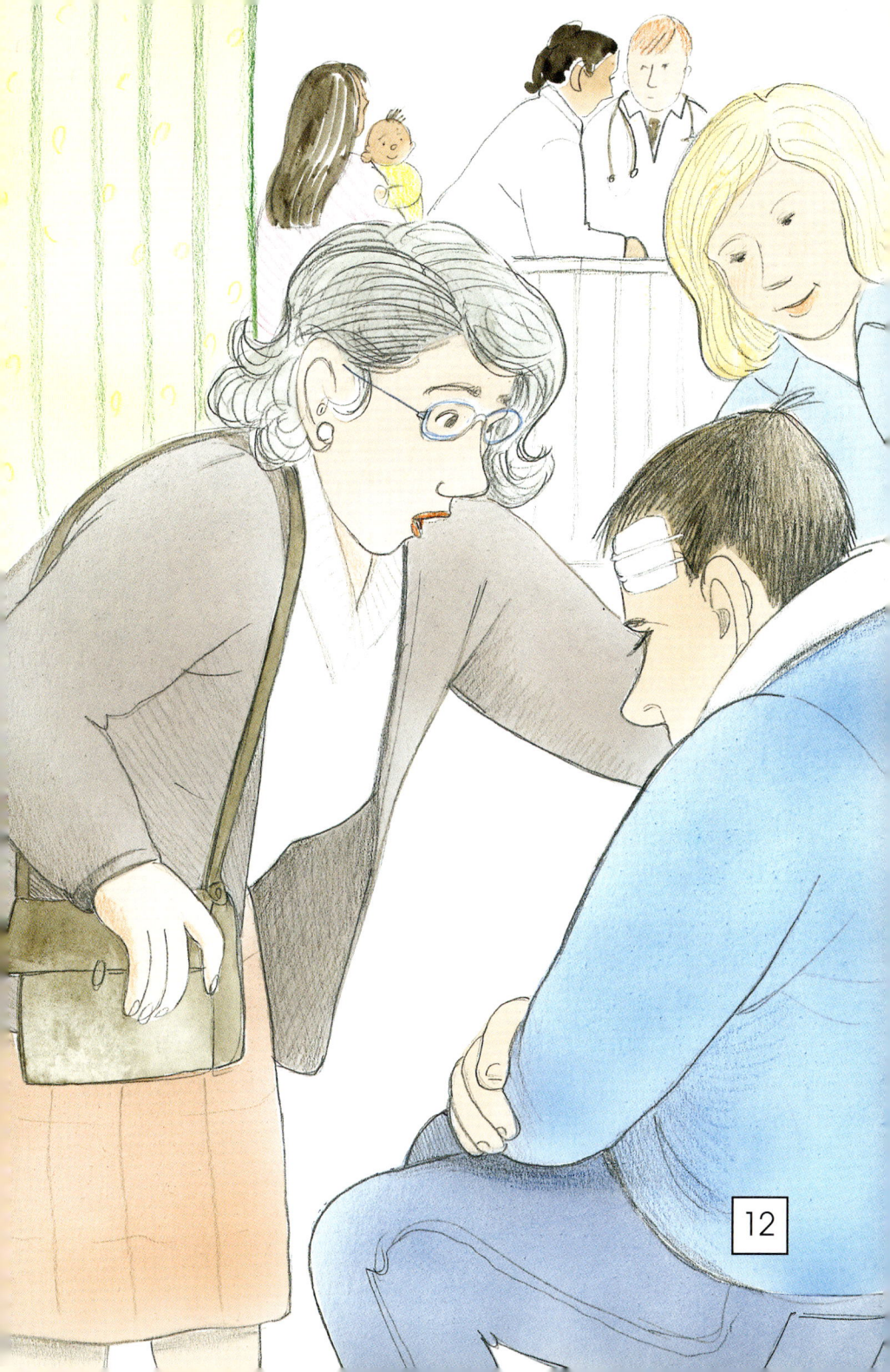

13

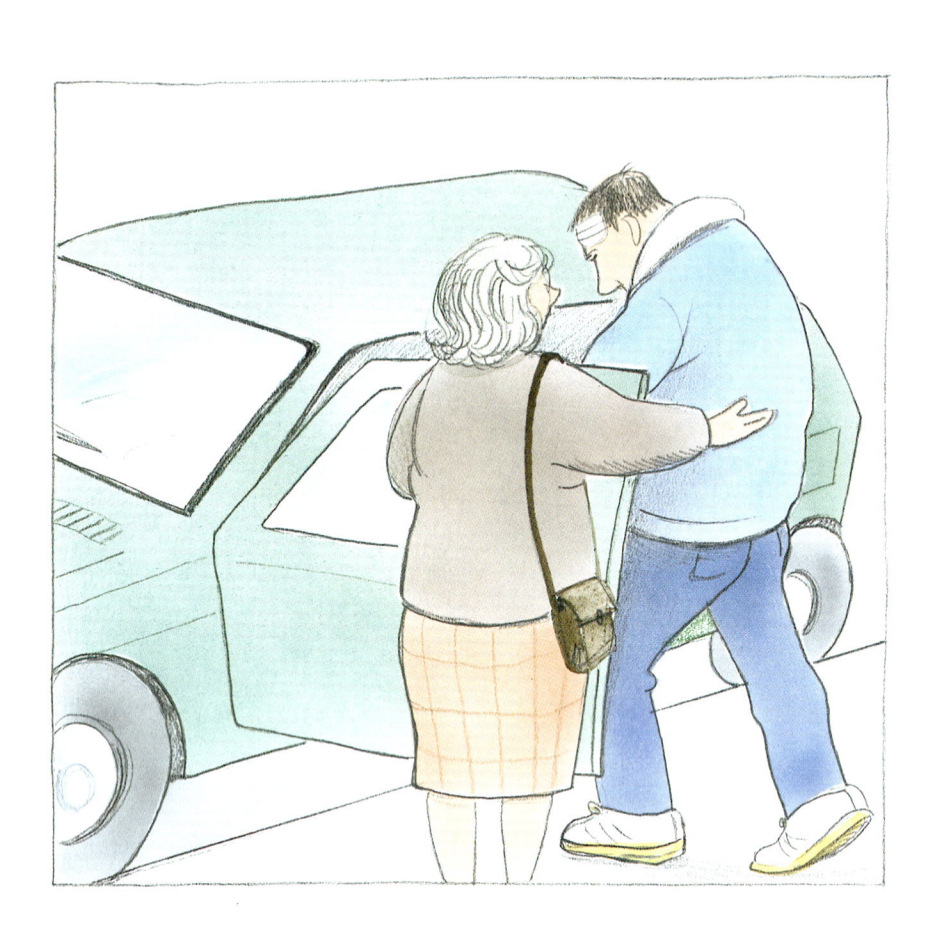

14

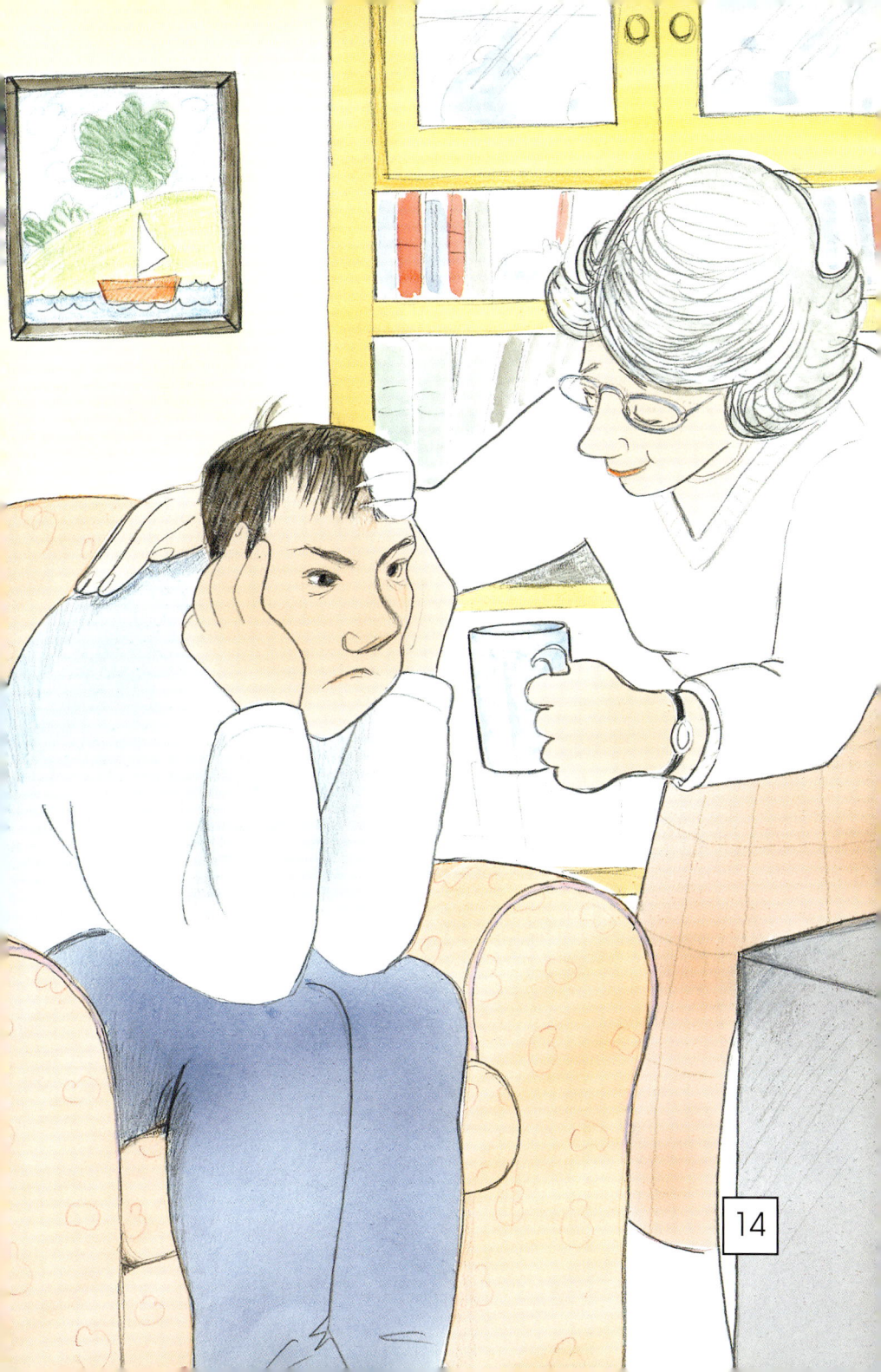

15

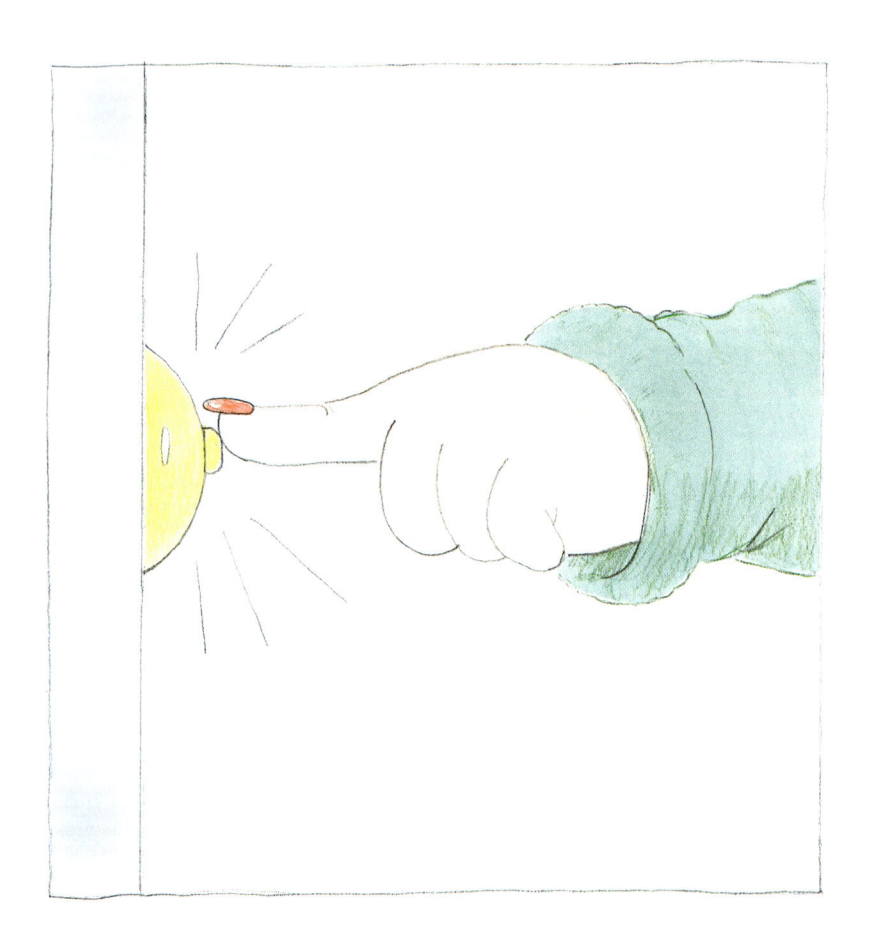

16

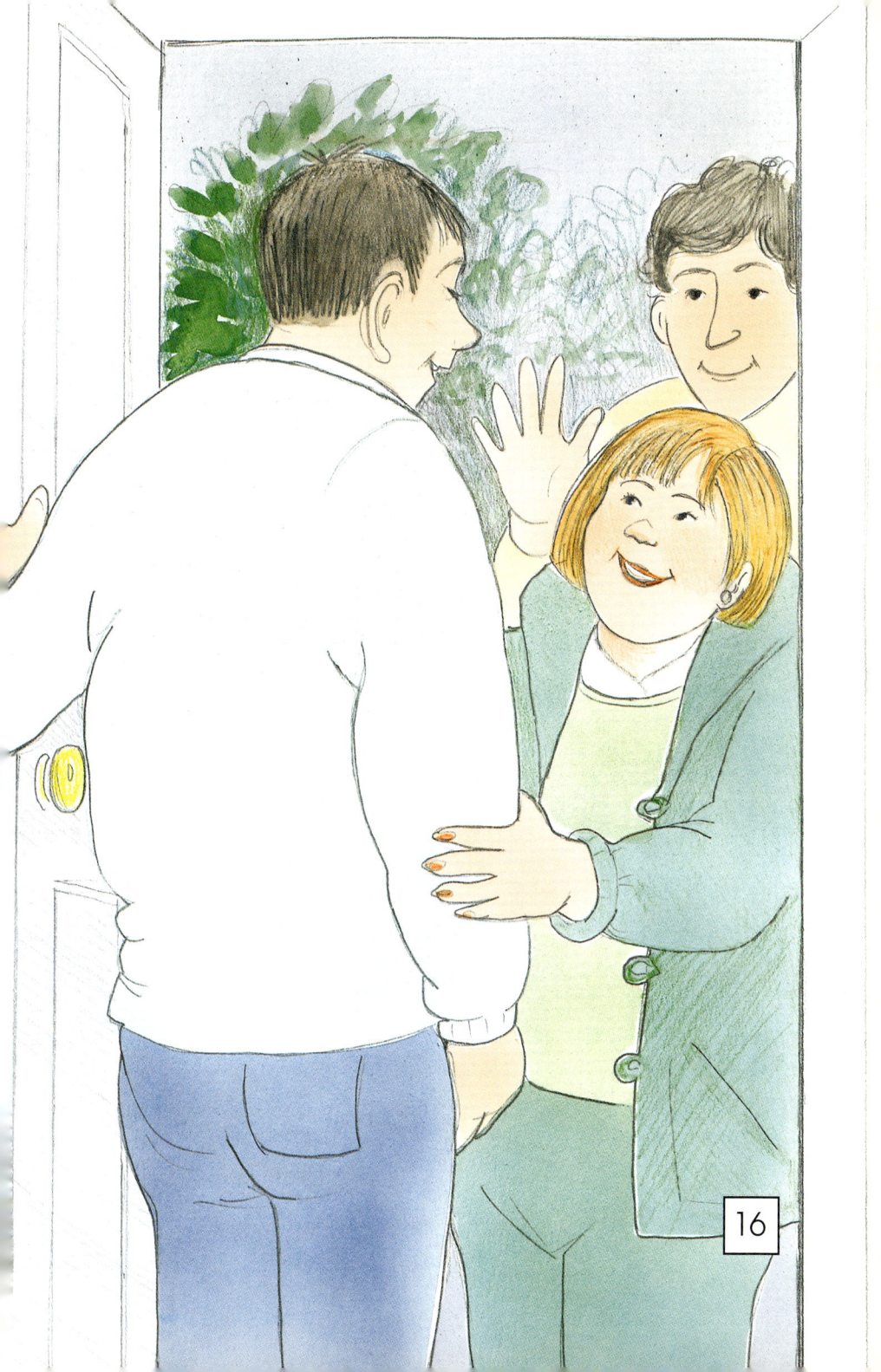

17

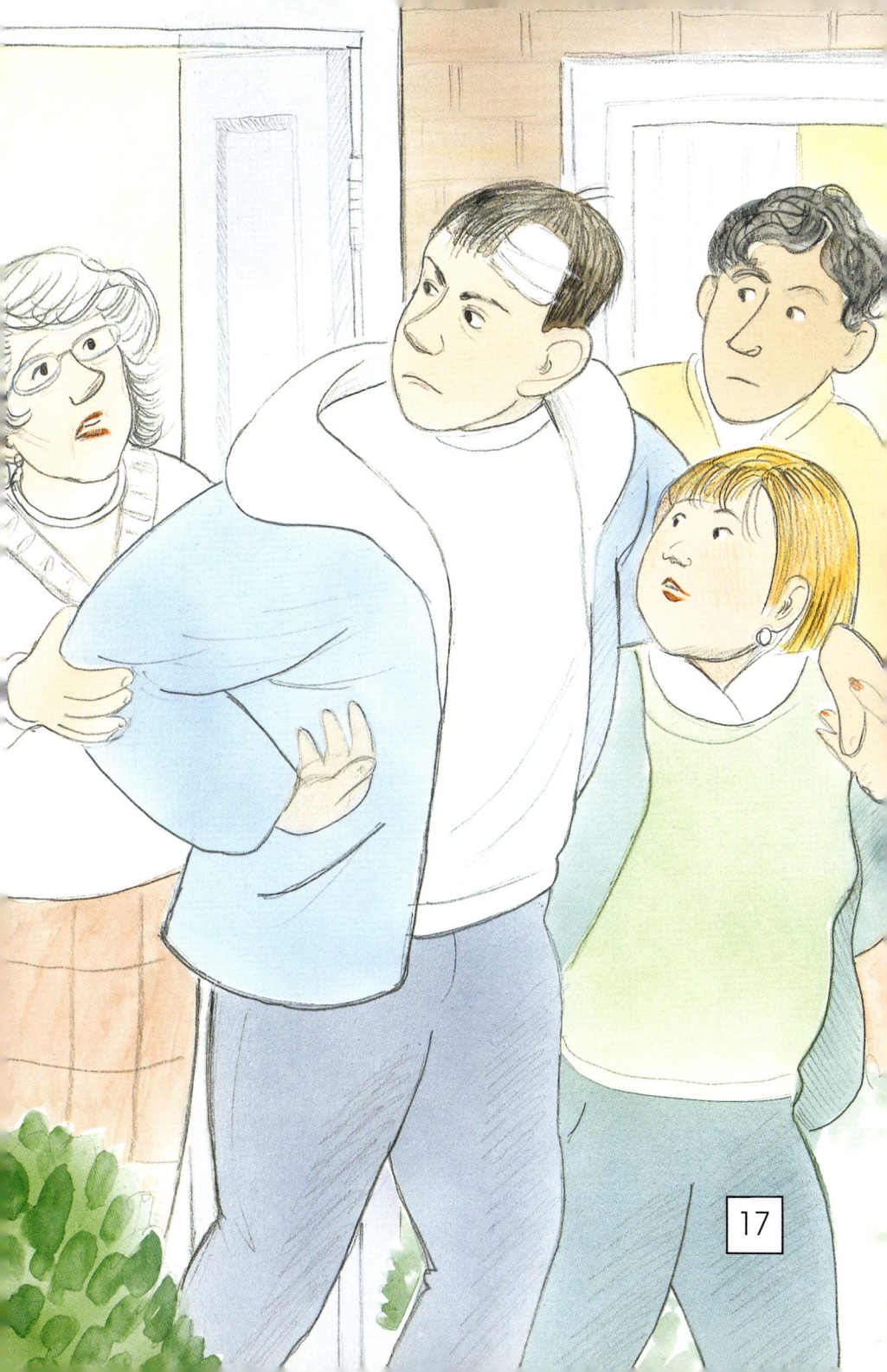

18

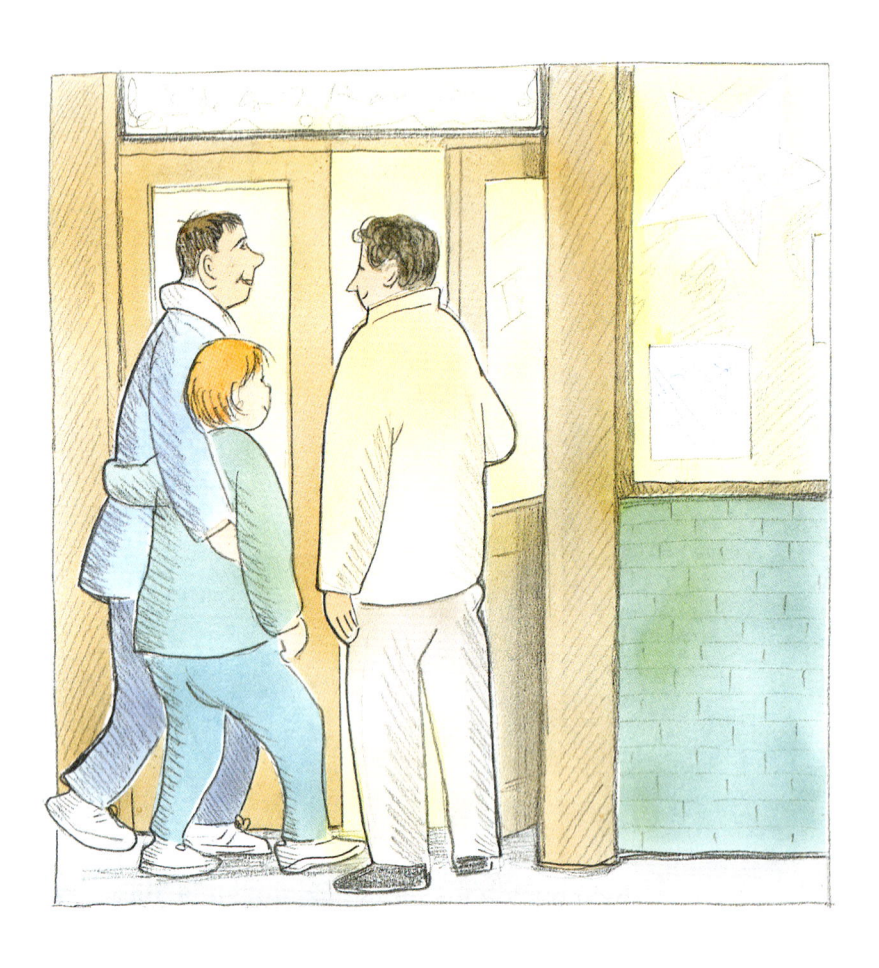

19

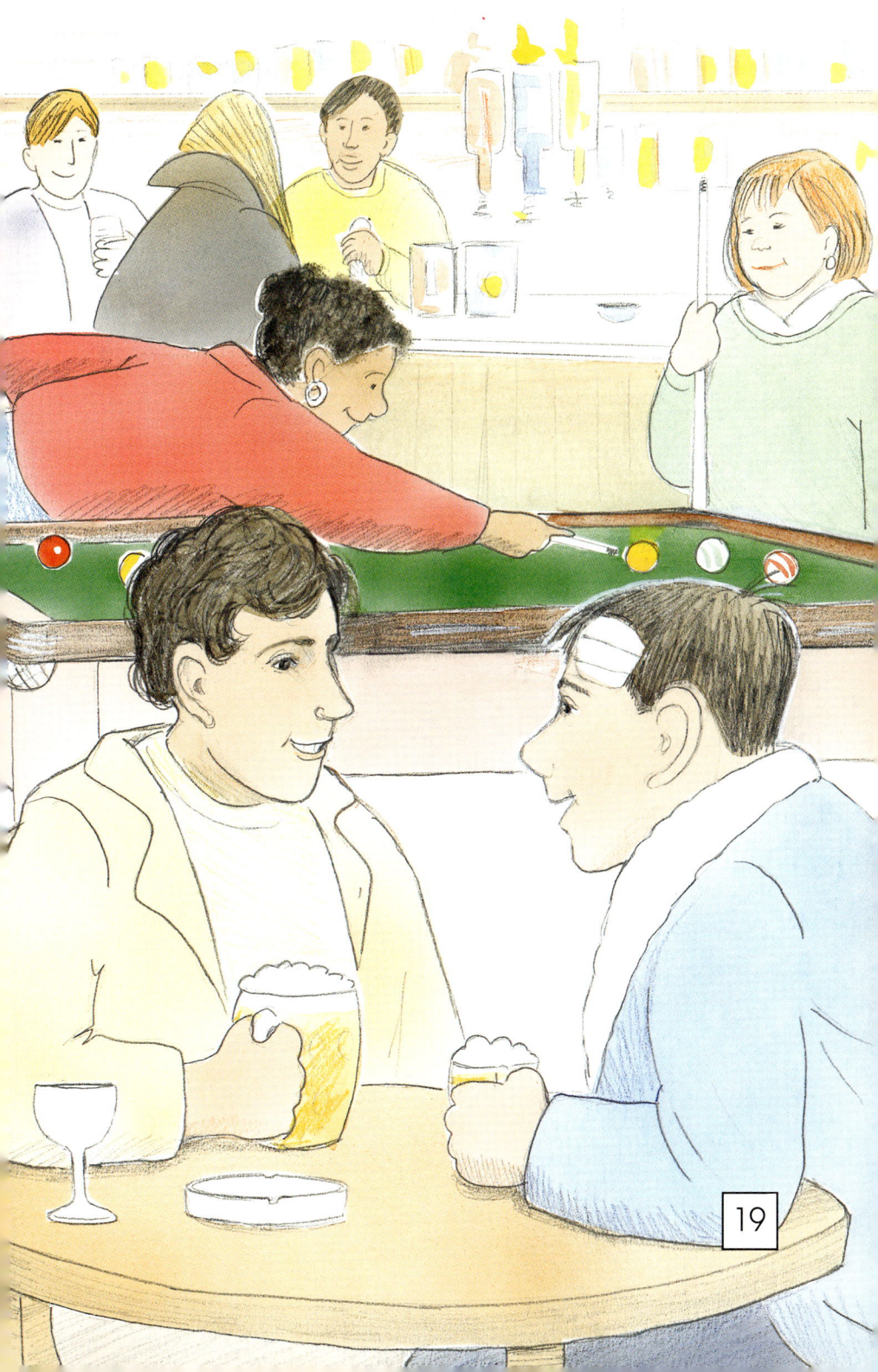

20

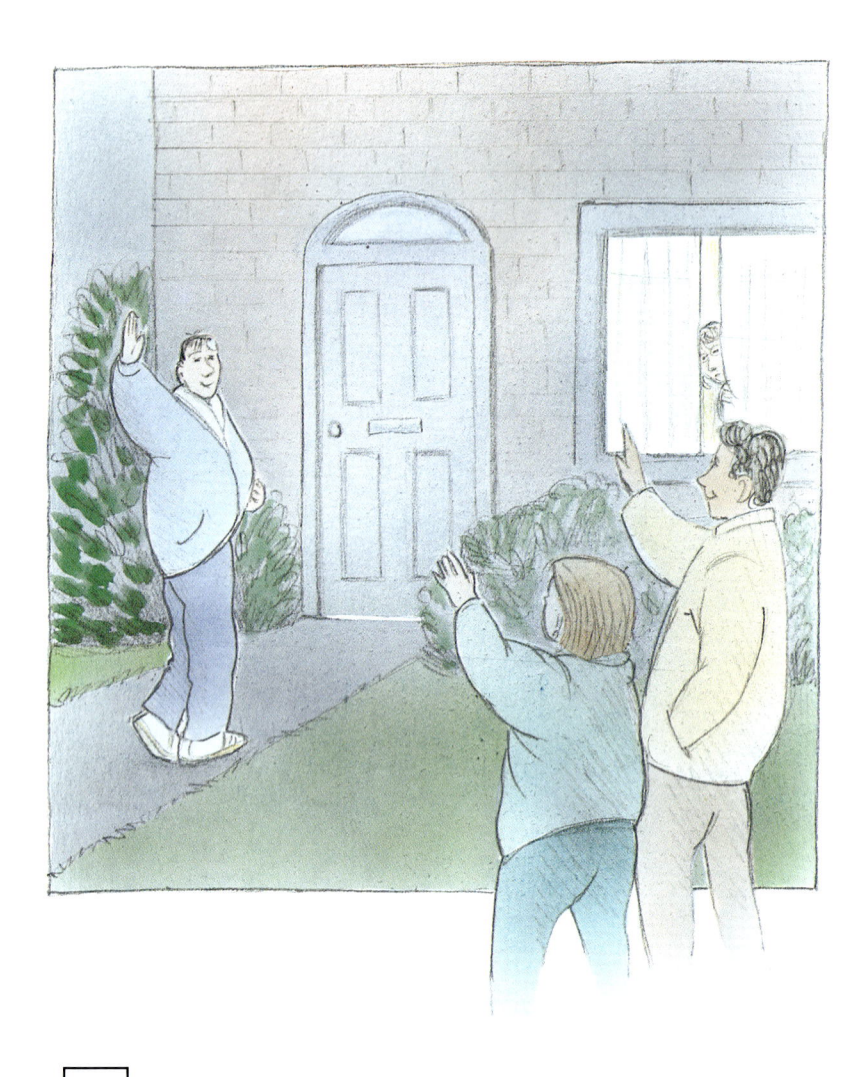

21

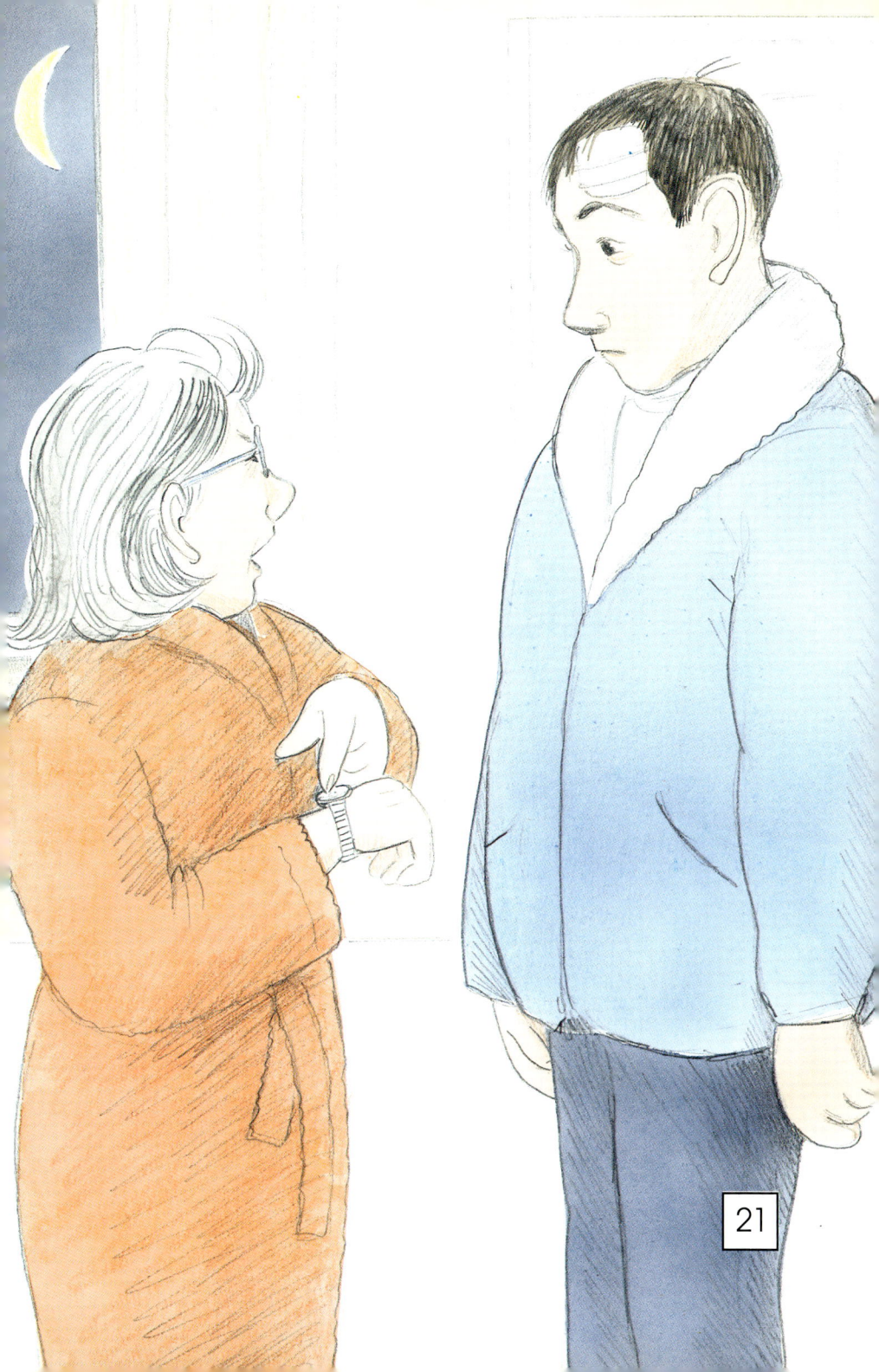

22

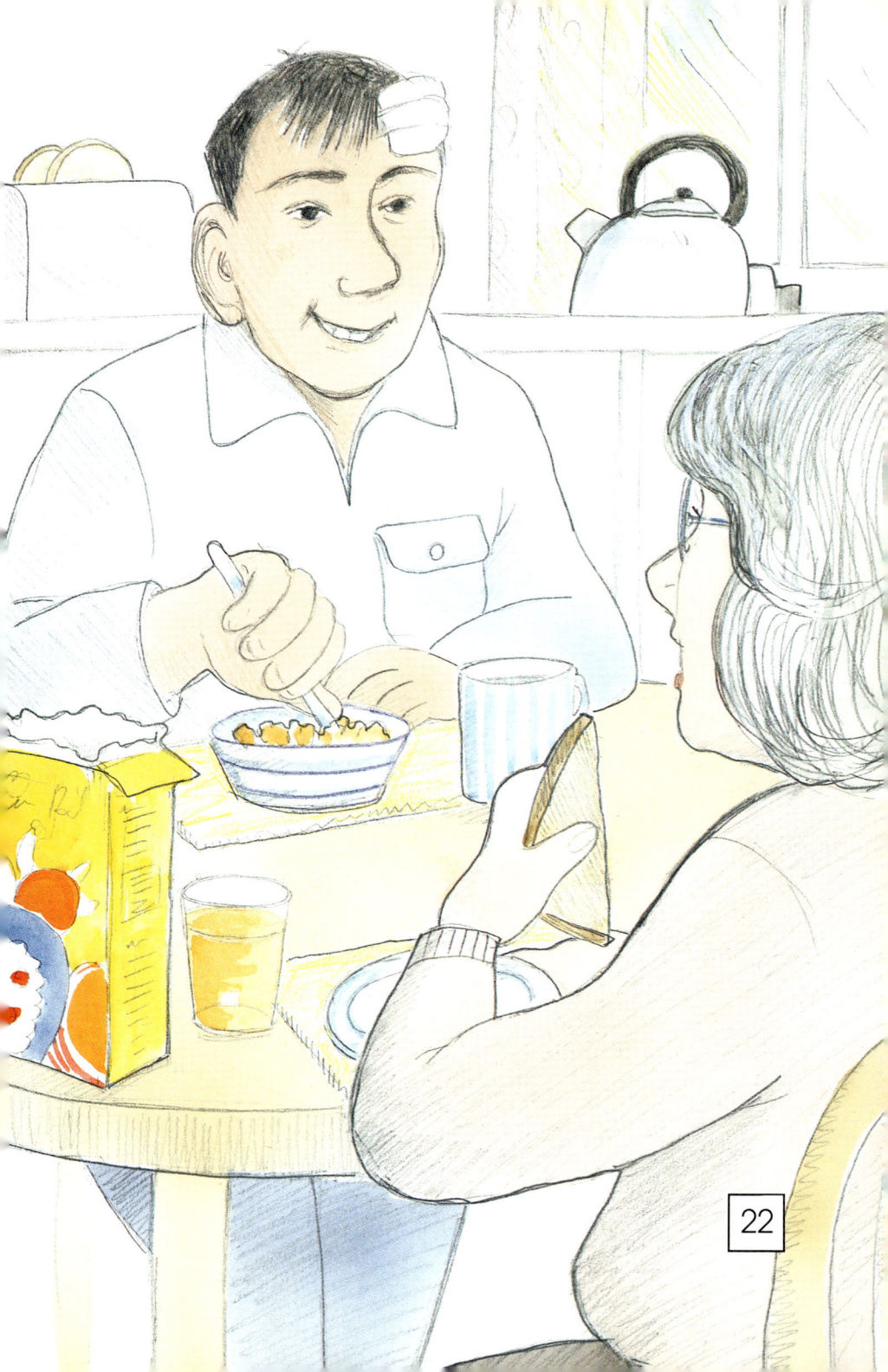

23

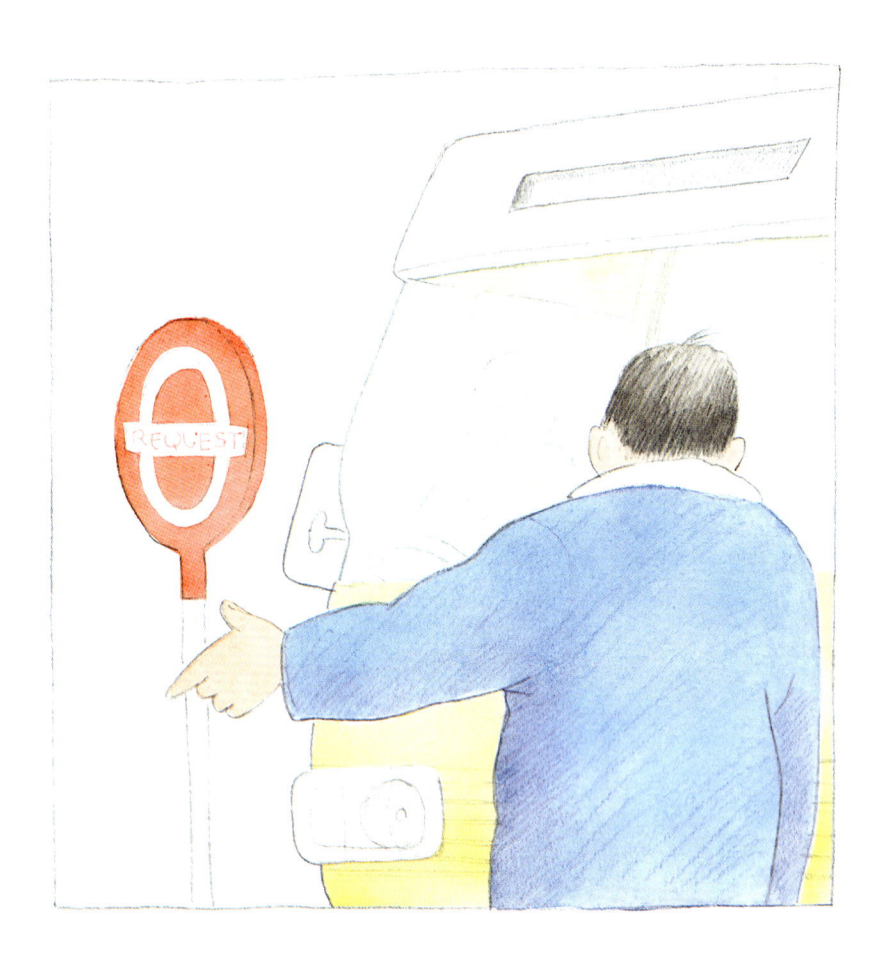

24

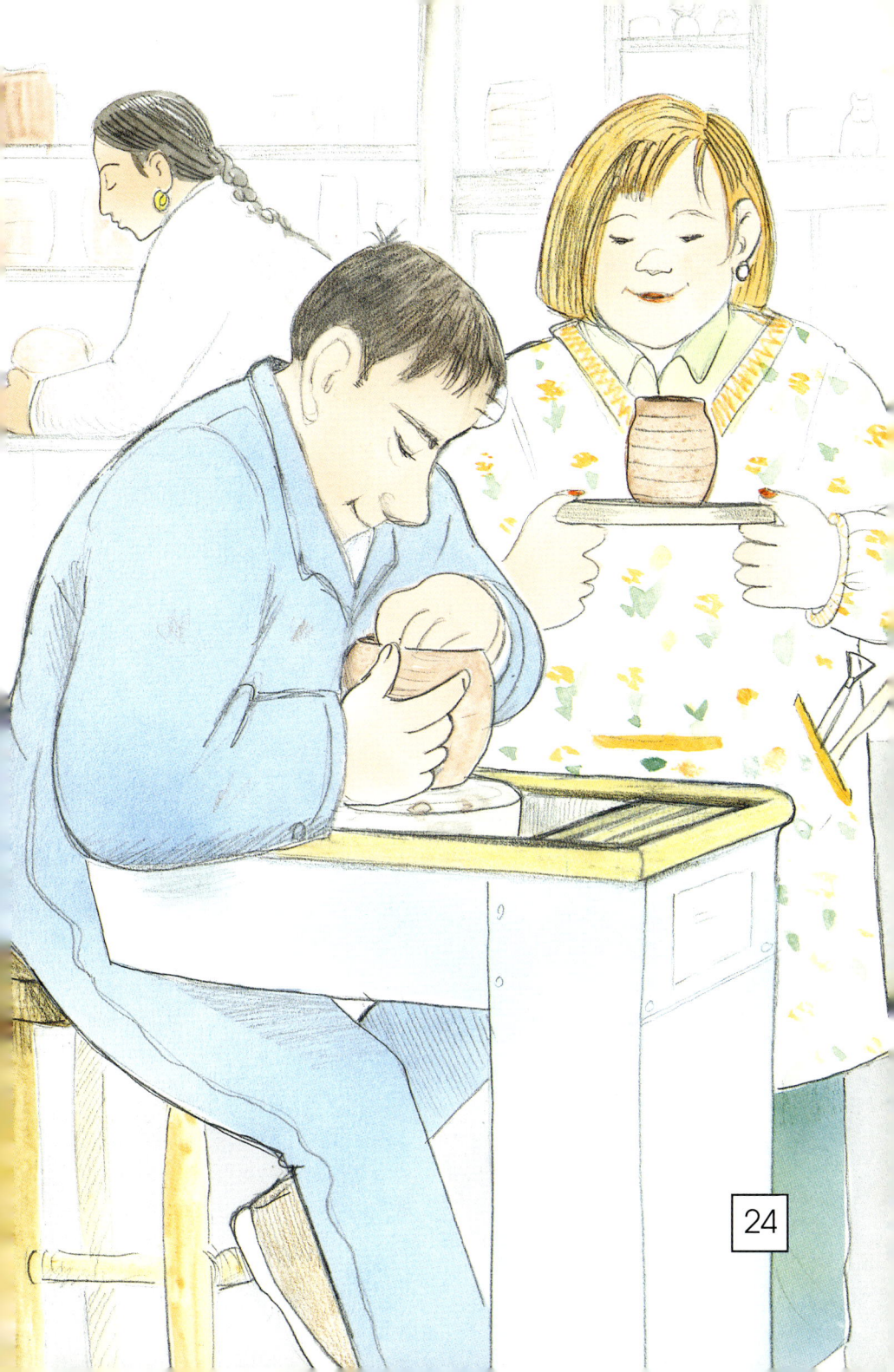

25

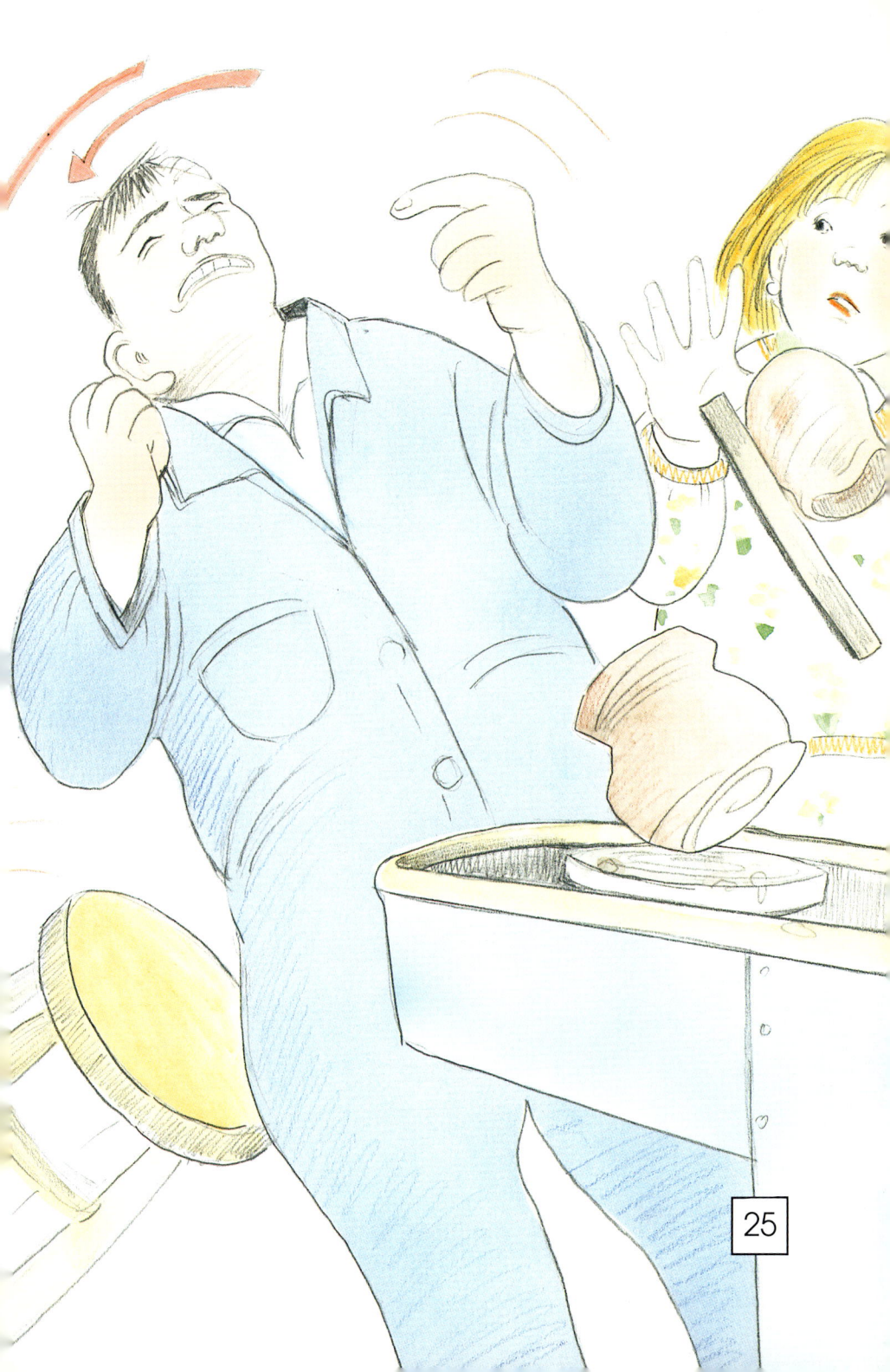

26

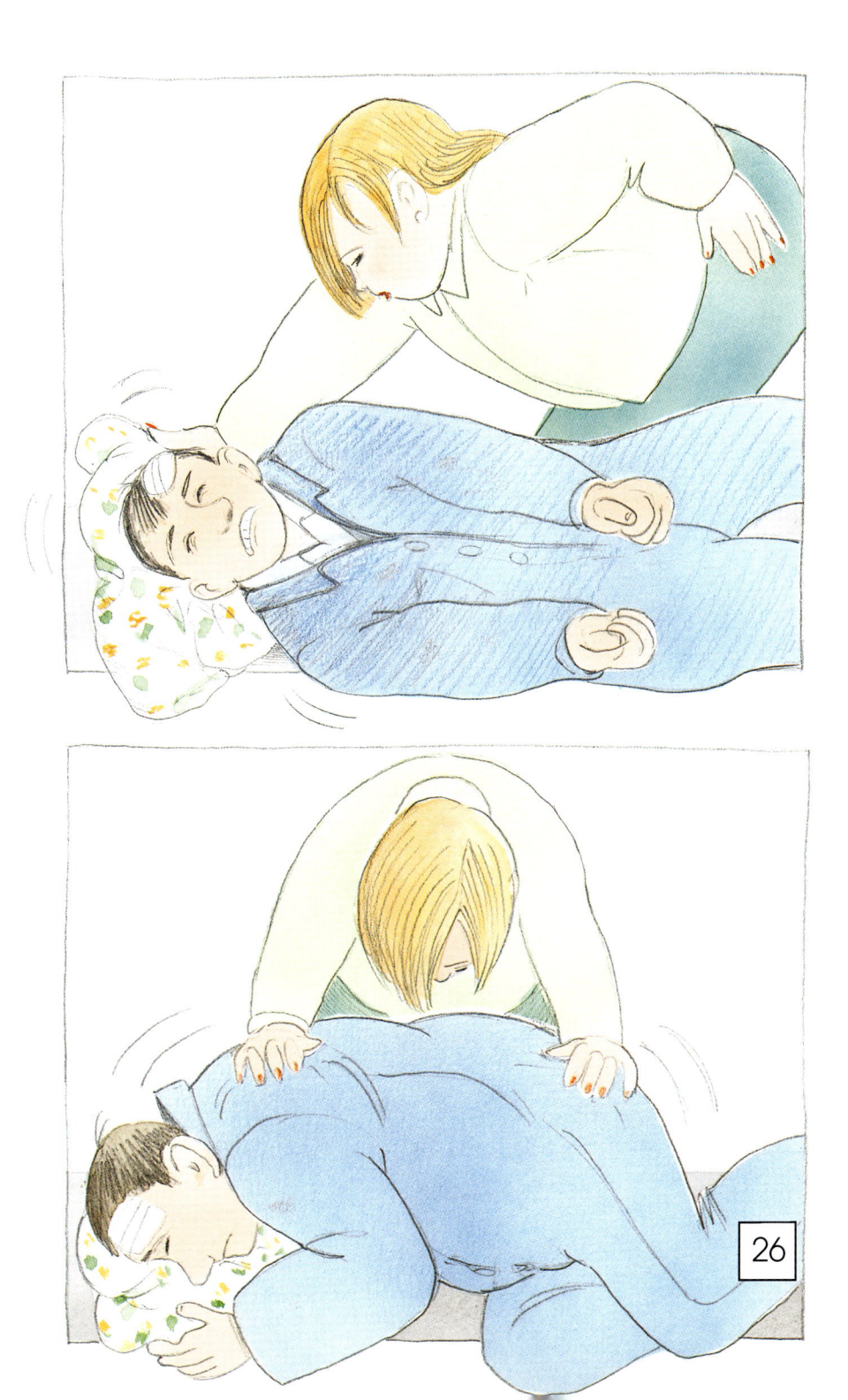

27

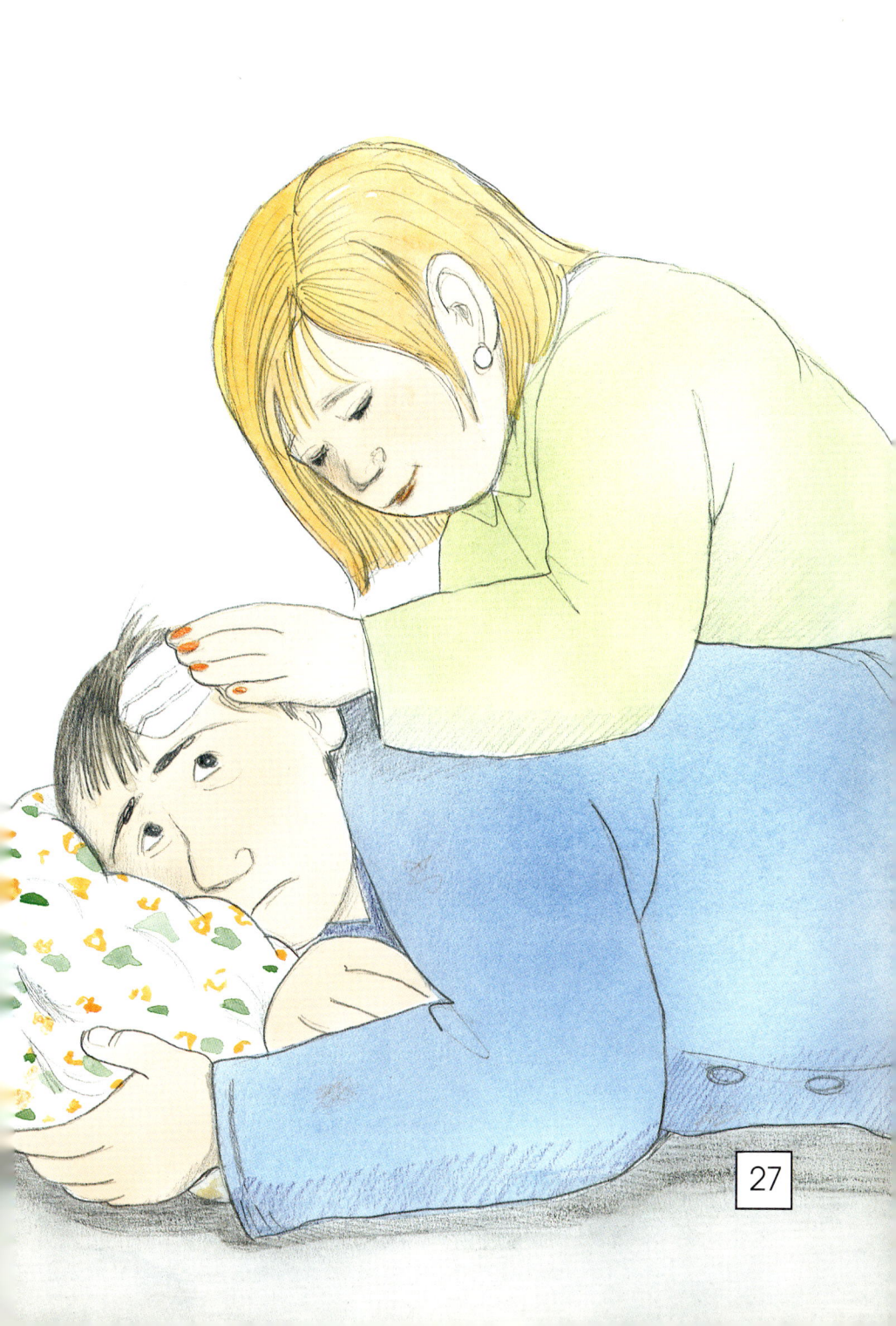

28

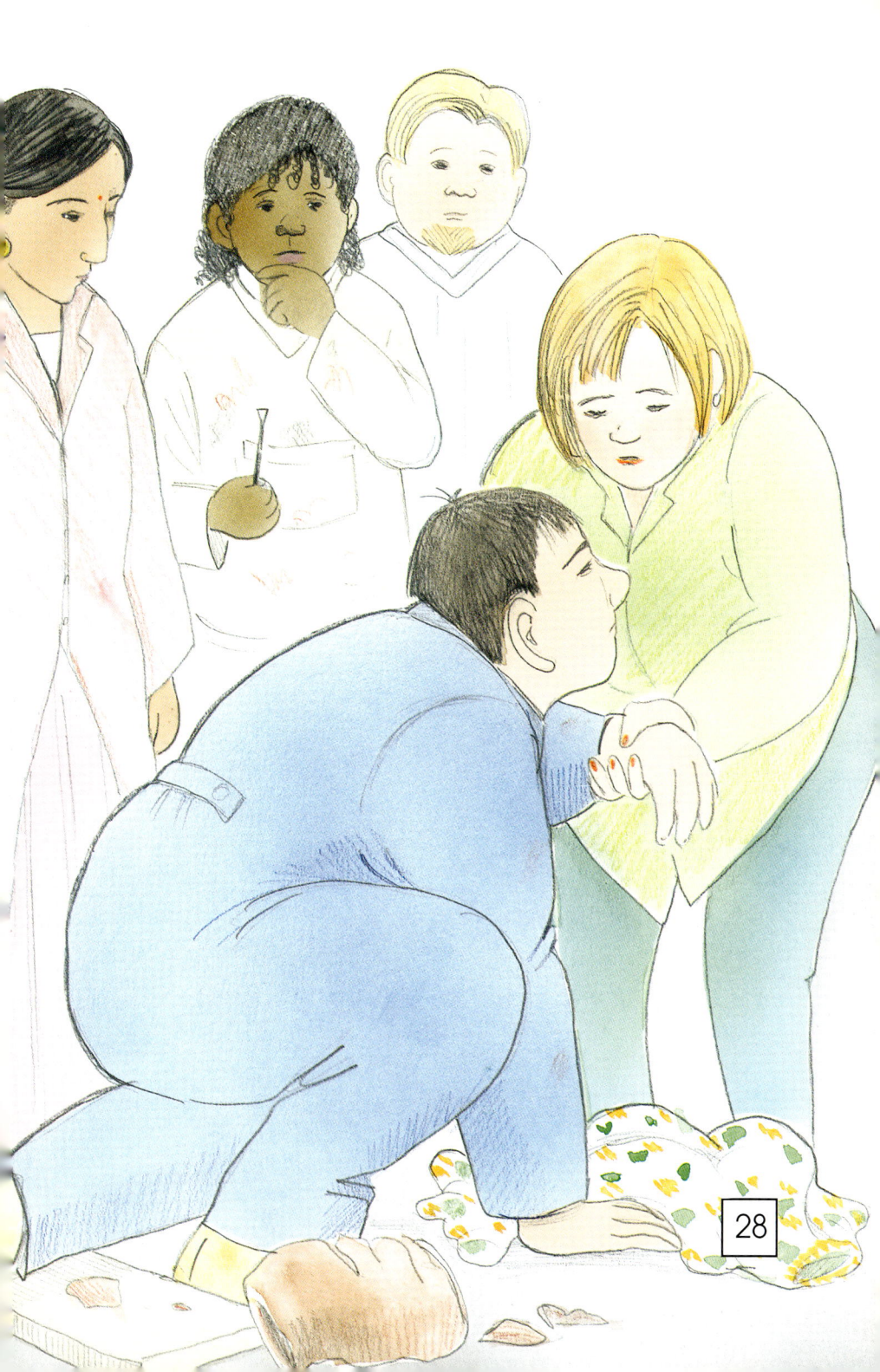

29

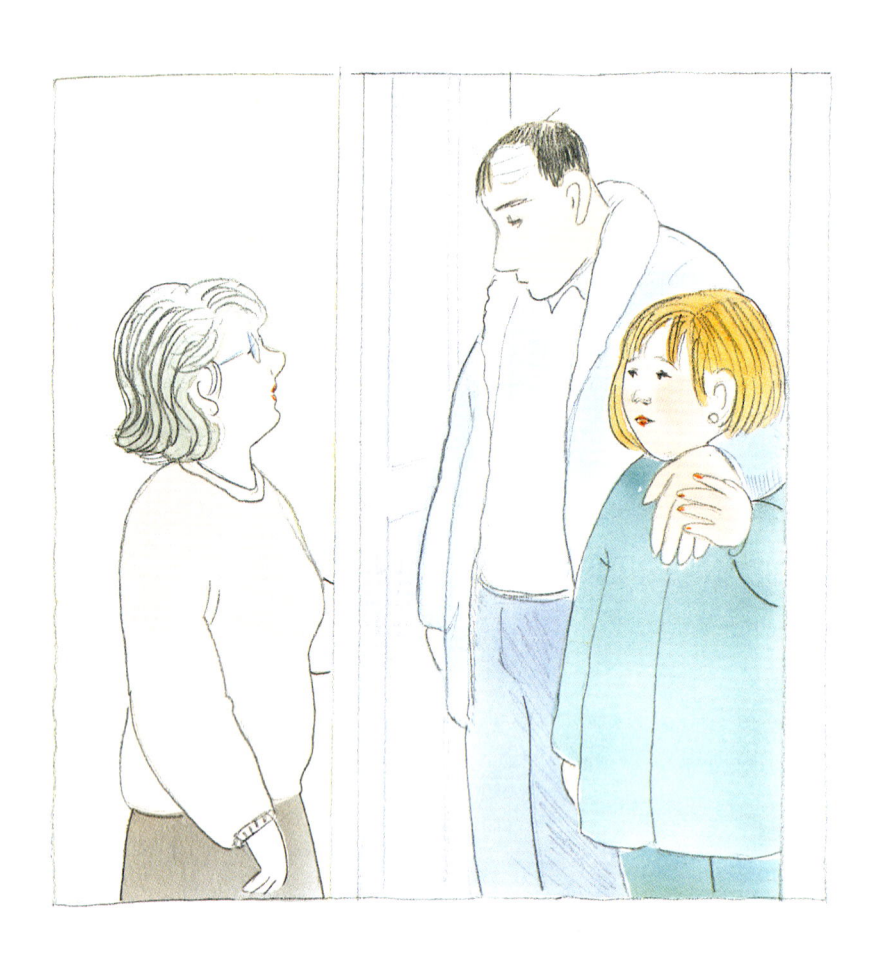

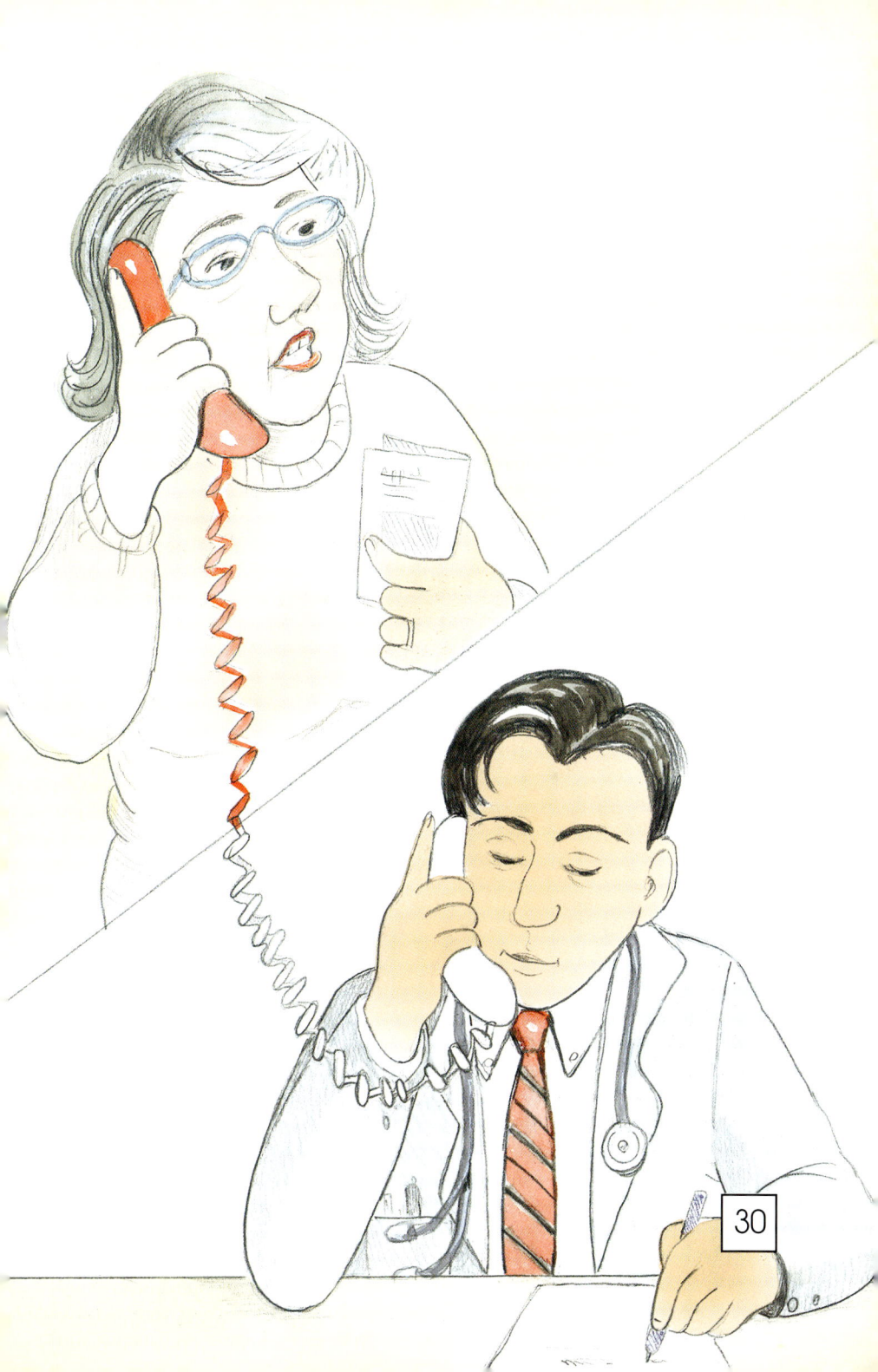

31

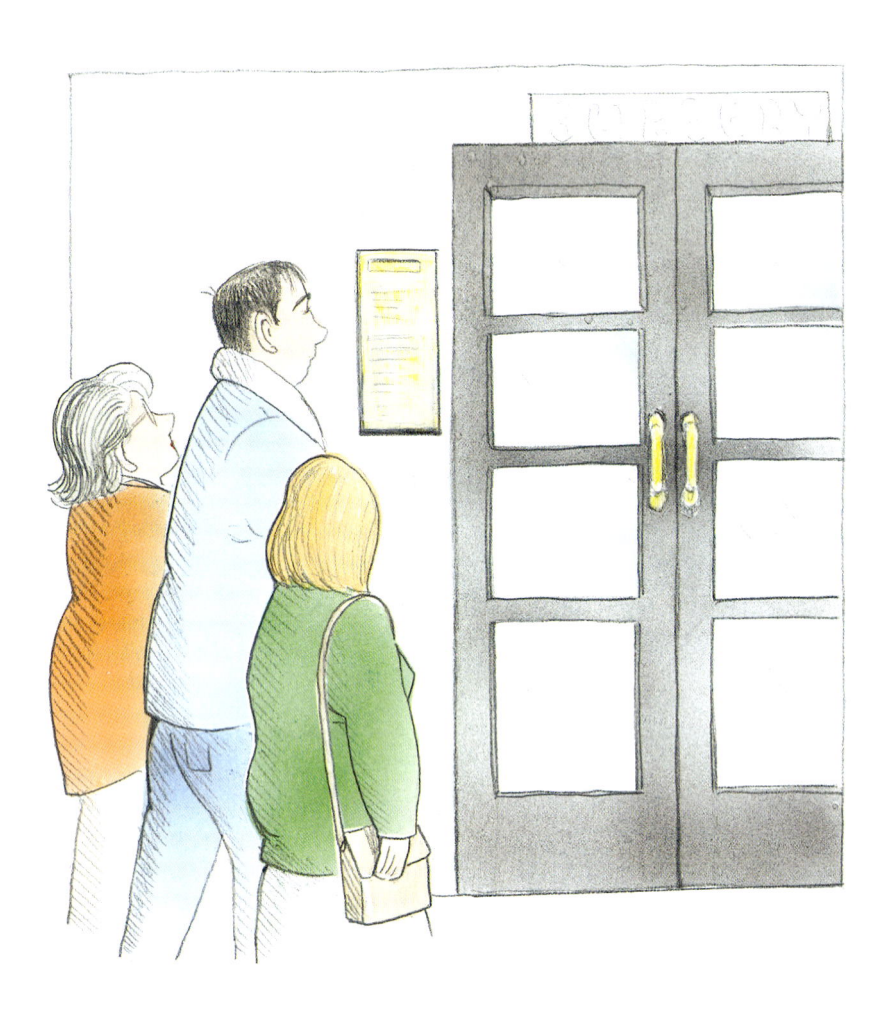

32

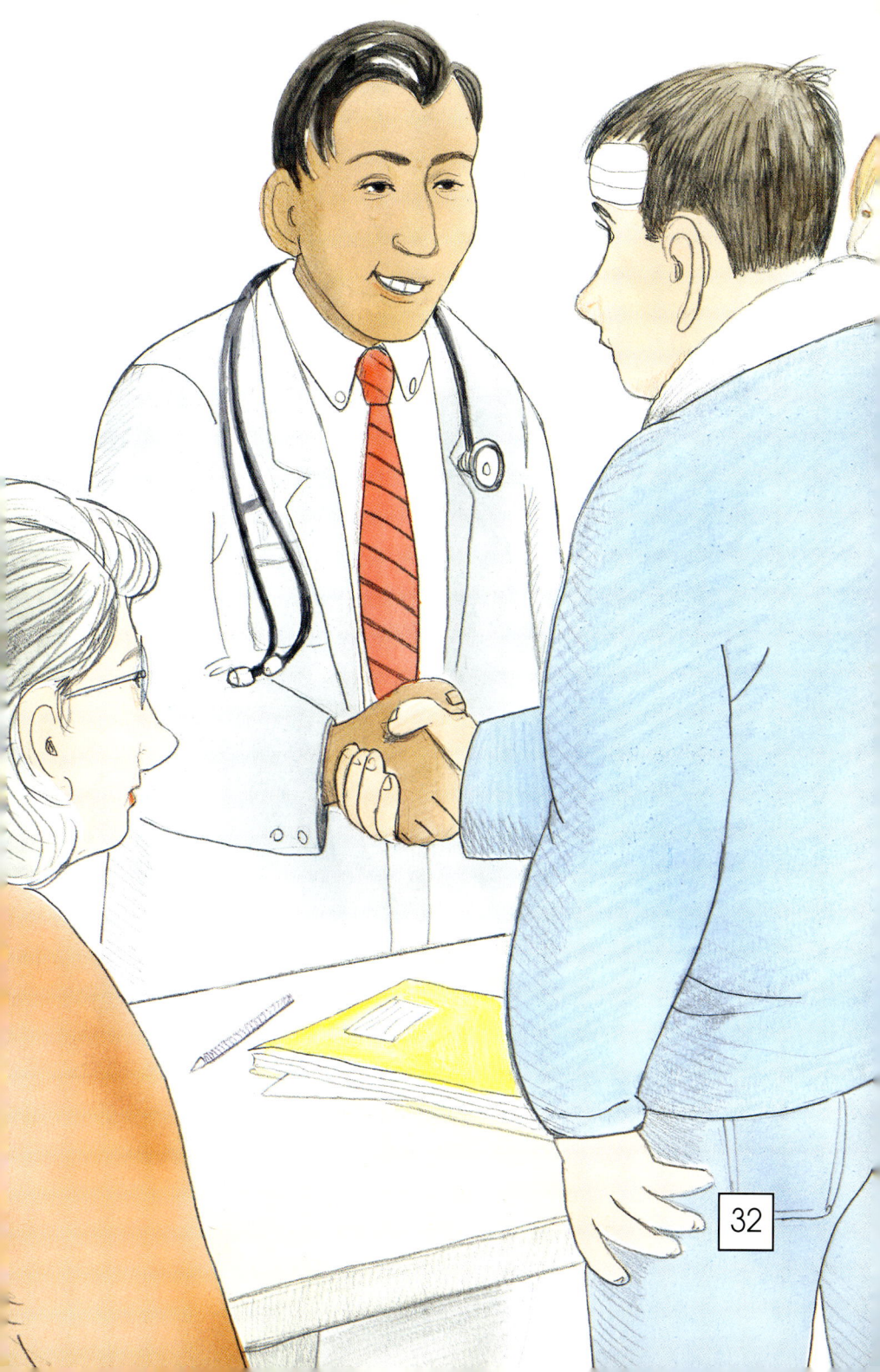

33

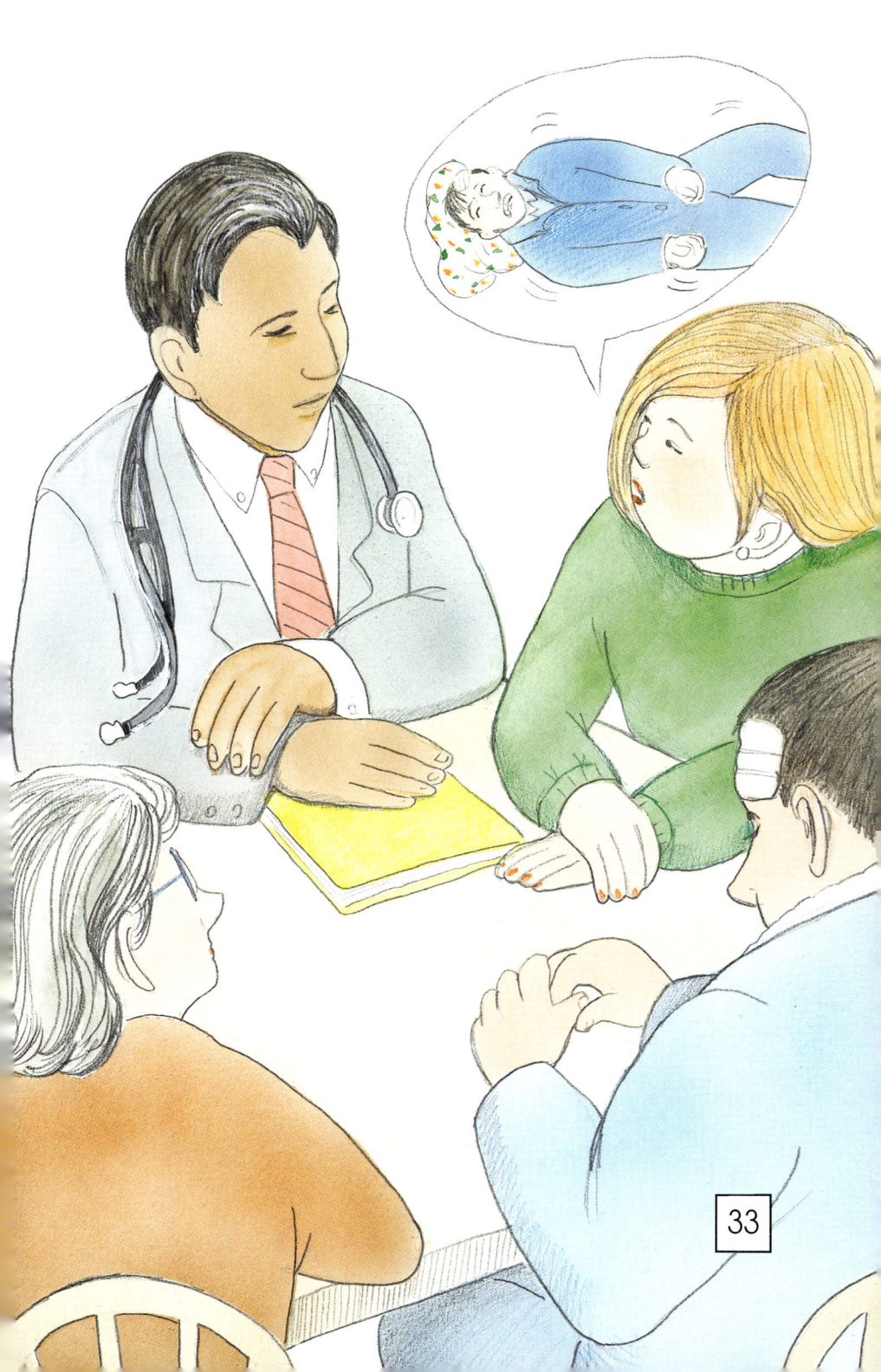

34

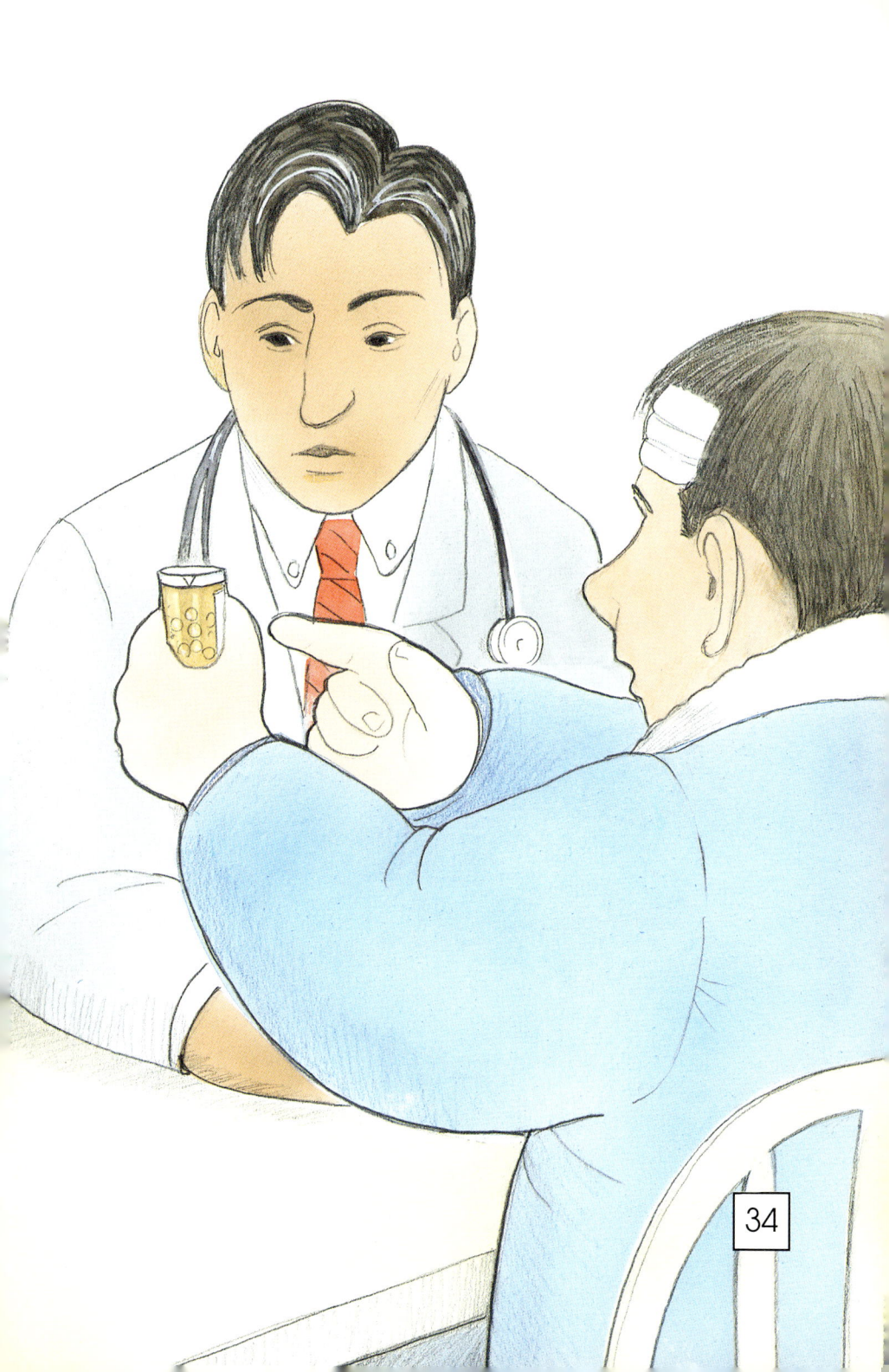

35

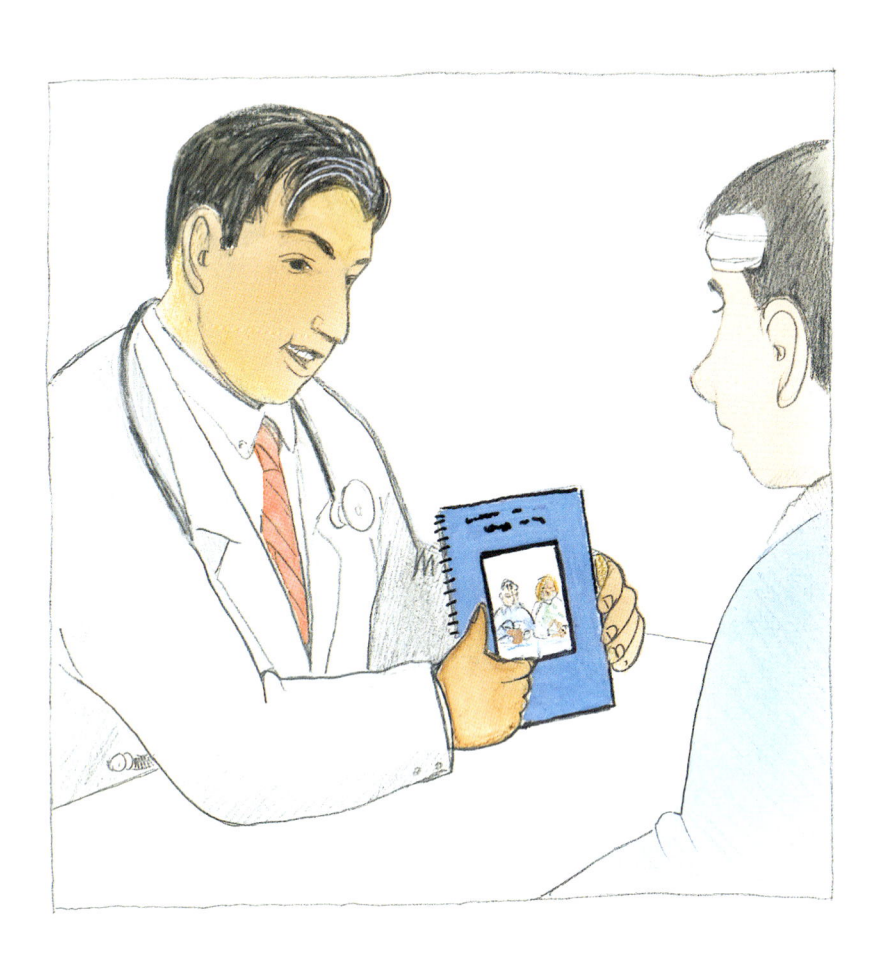

36

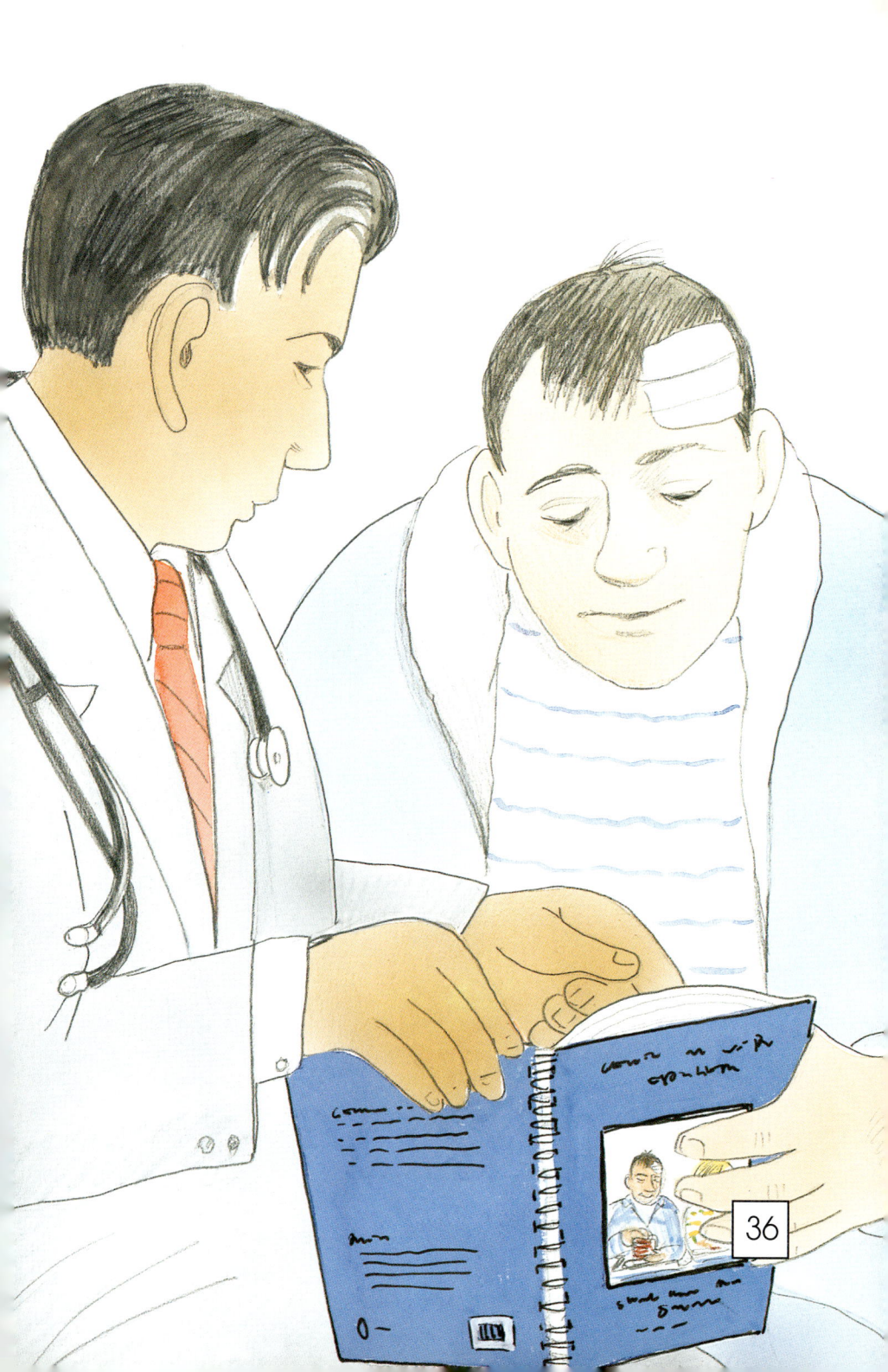

37

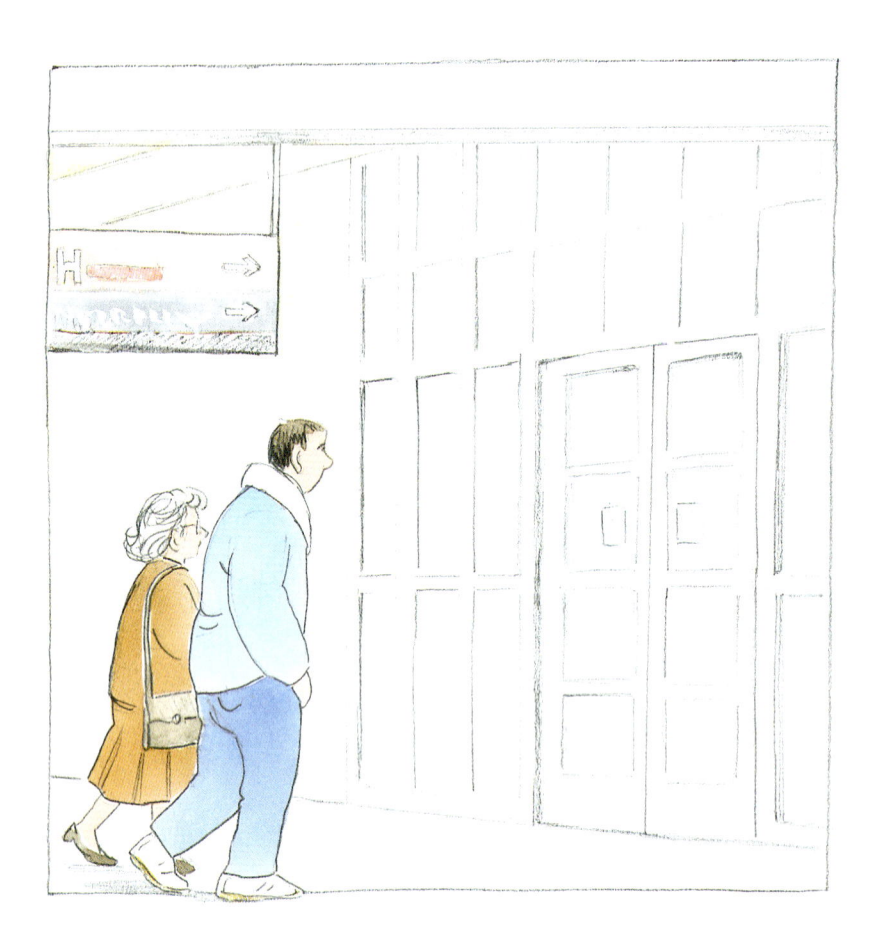

38

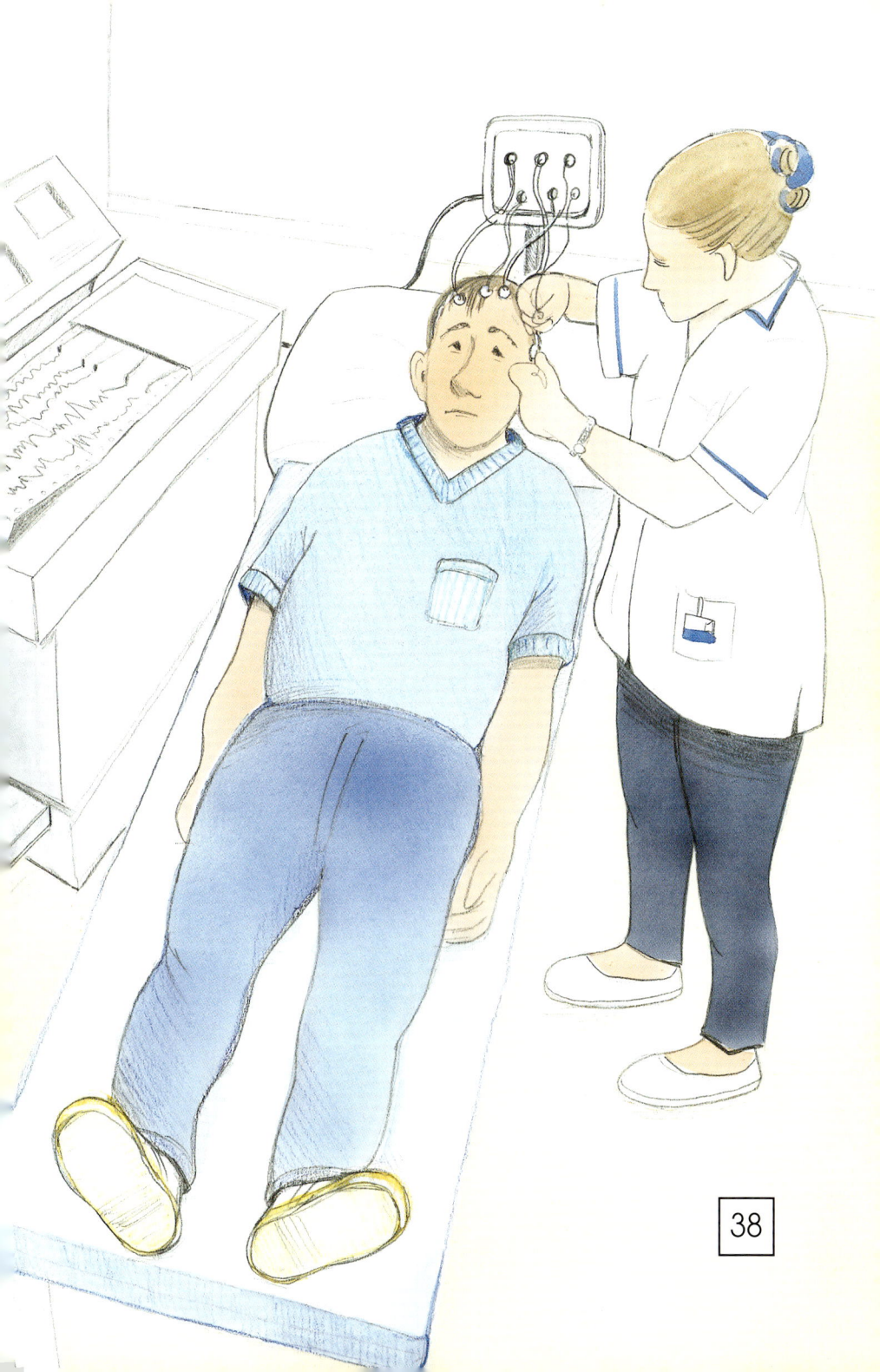

39

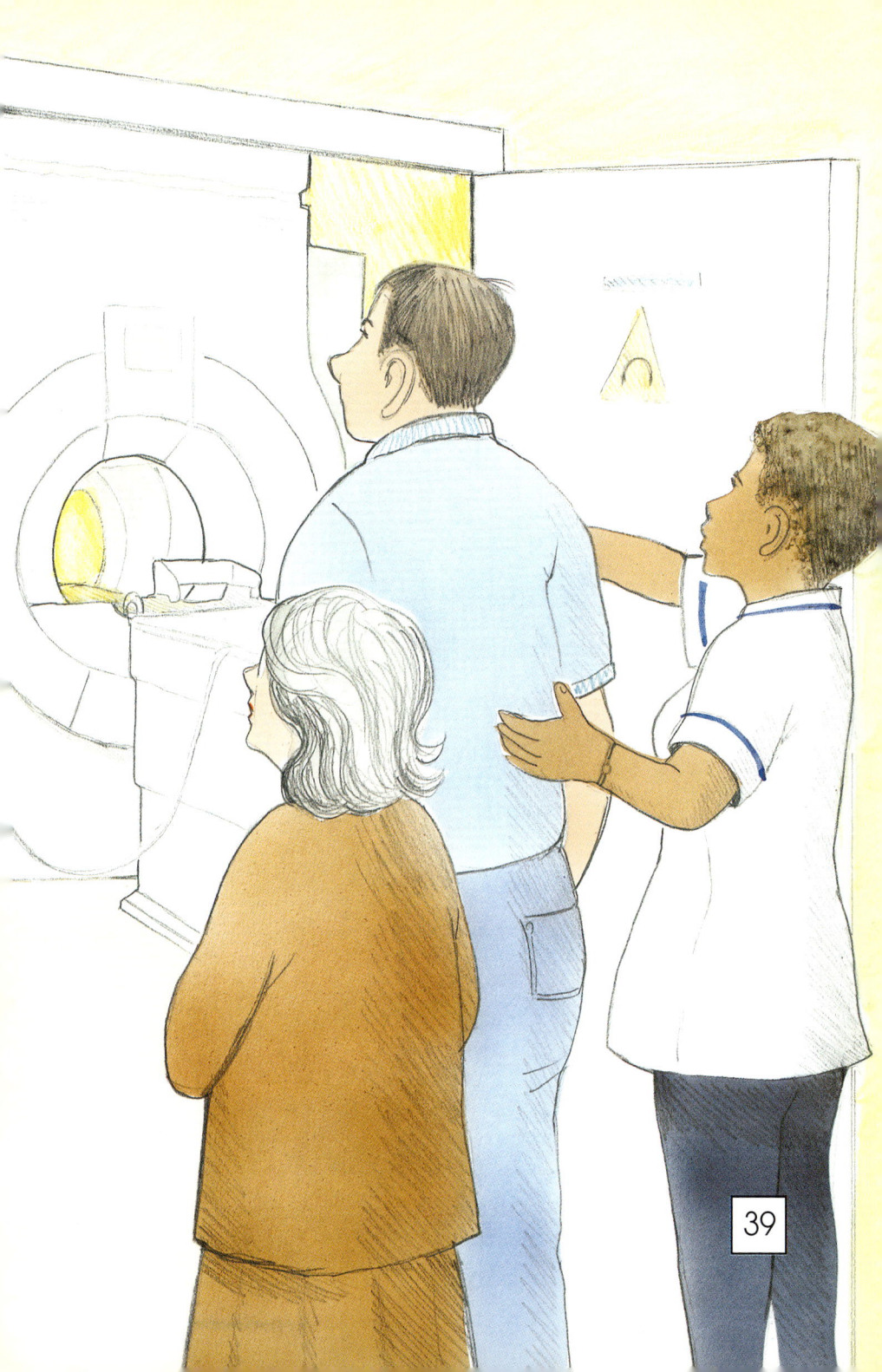

40

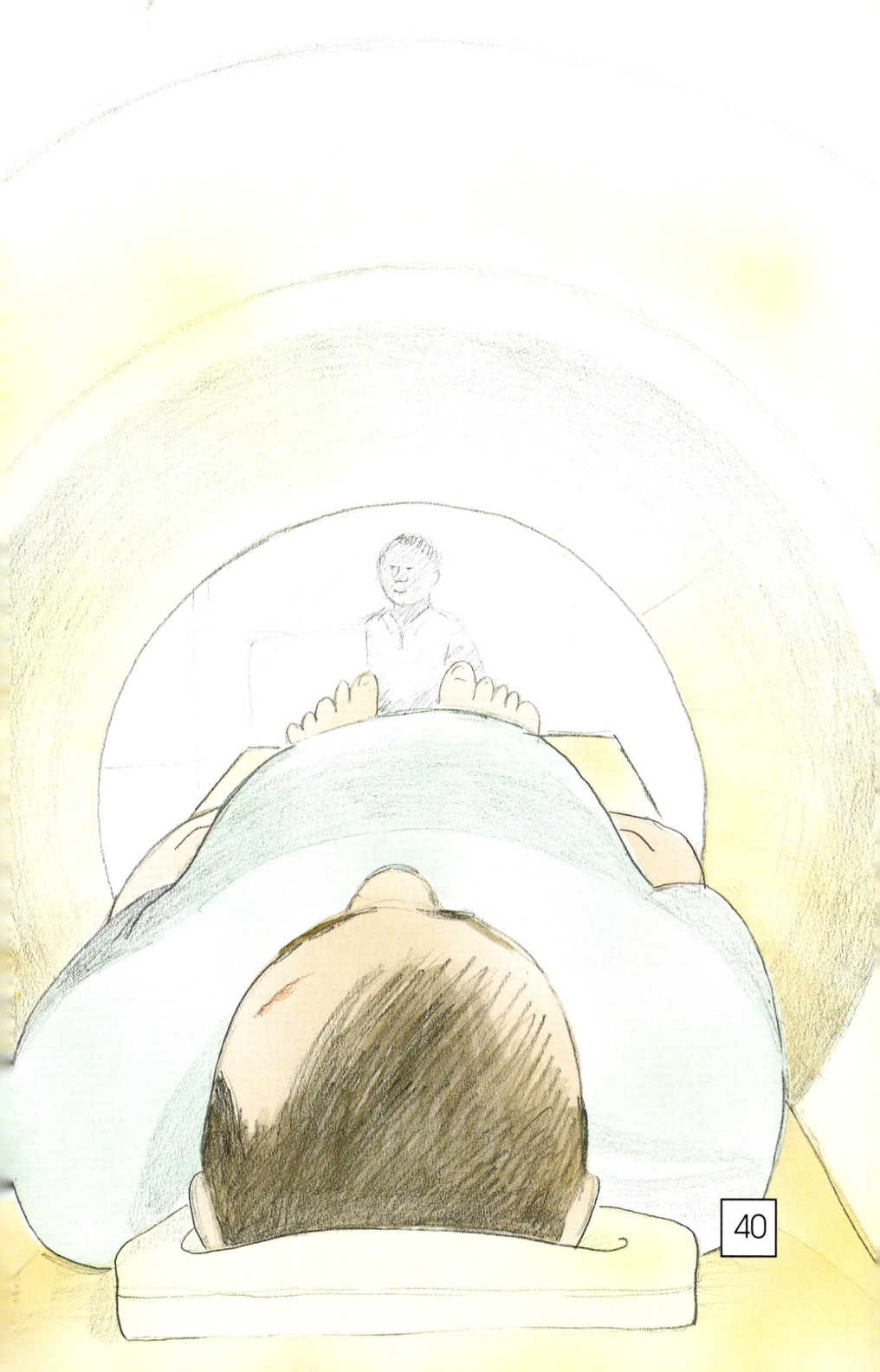

41

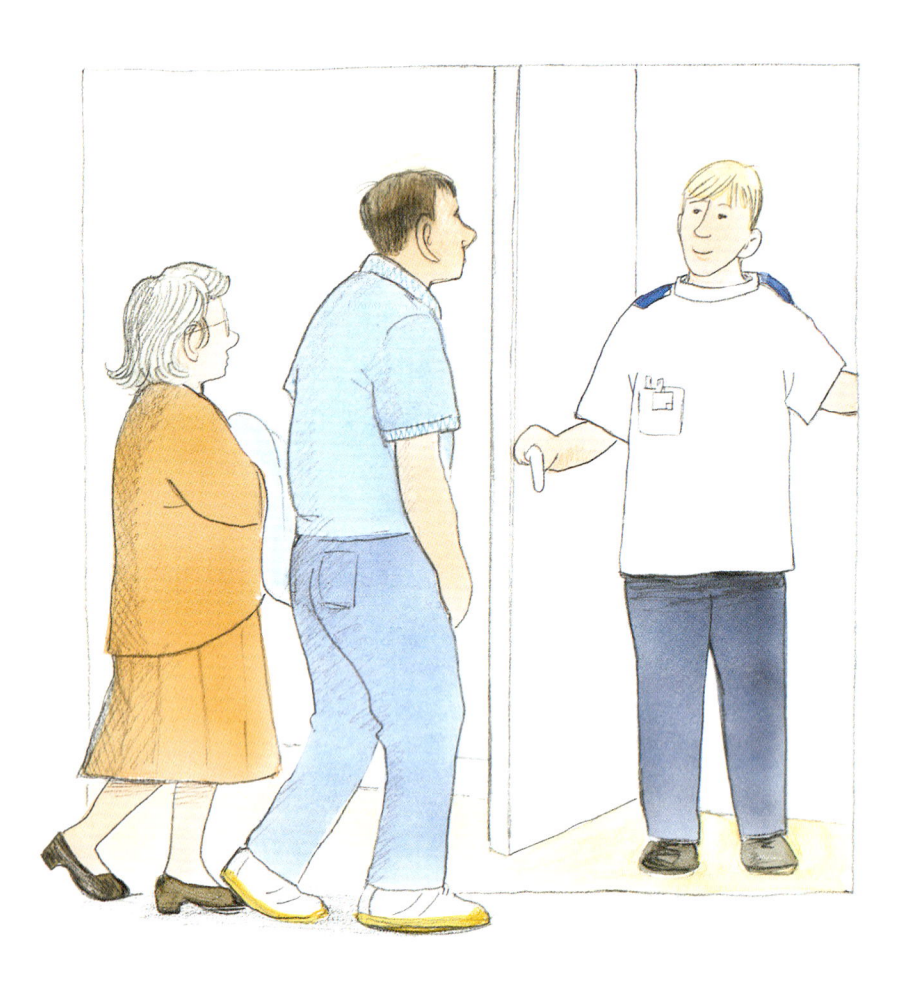

42

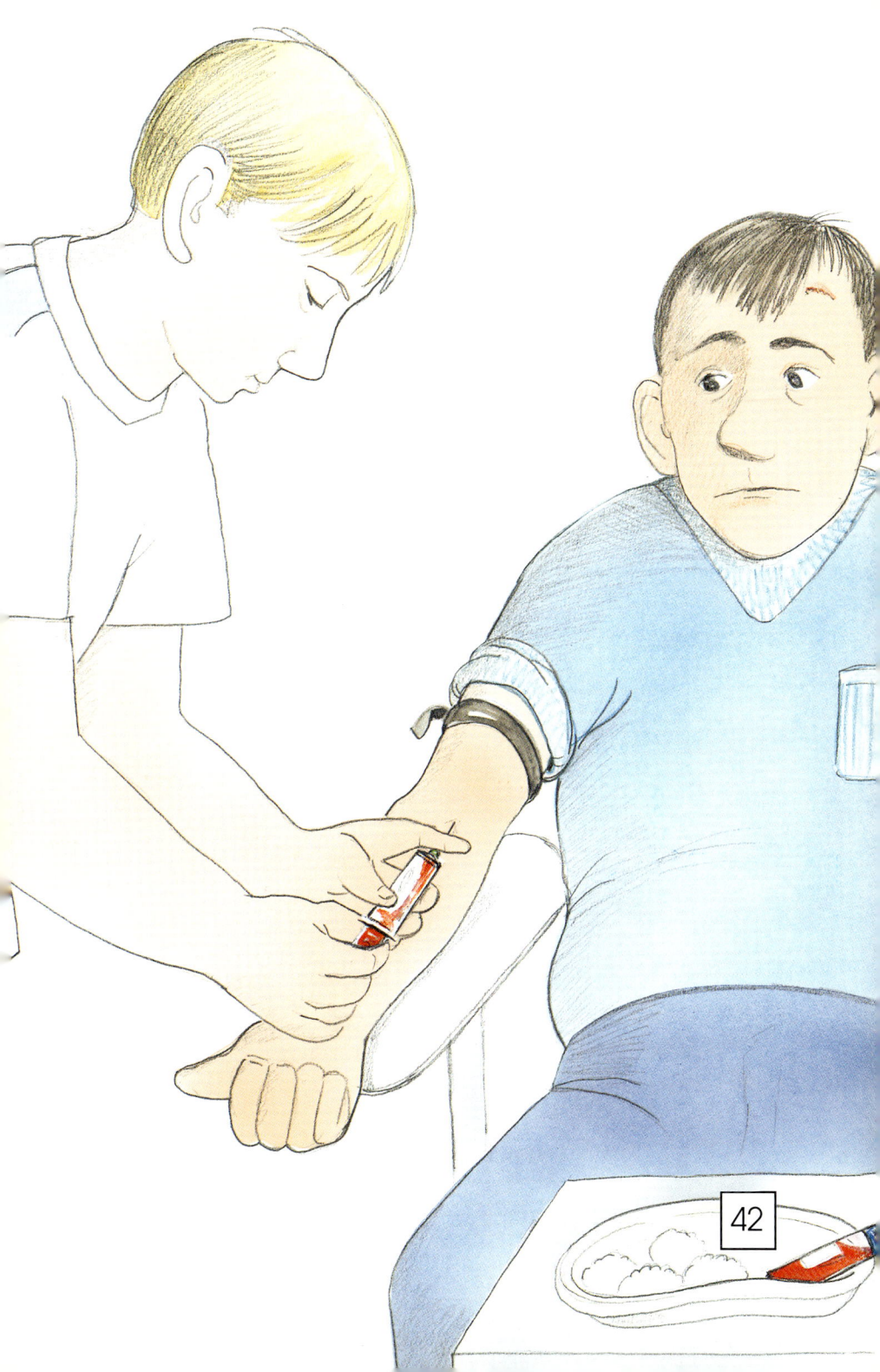

43

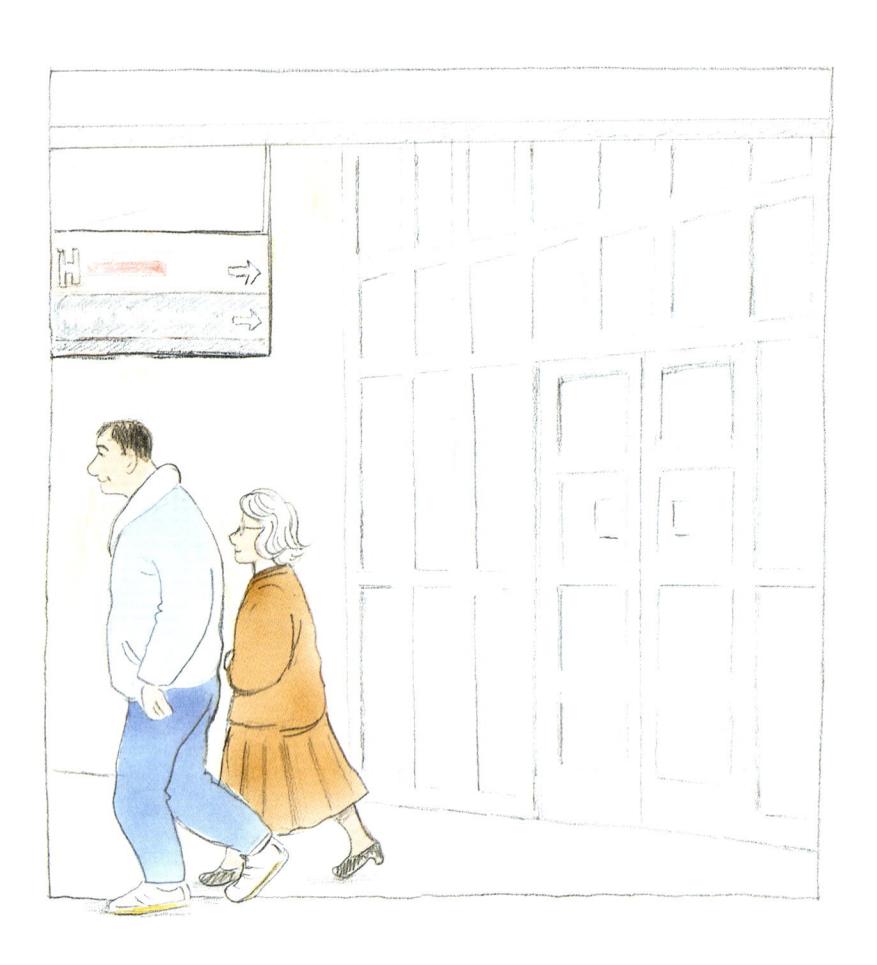

44

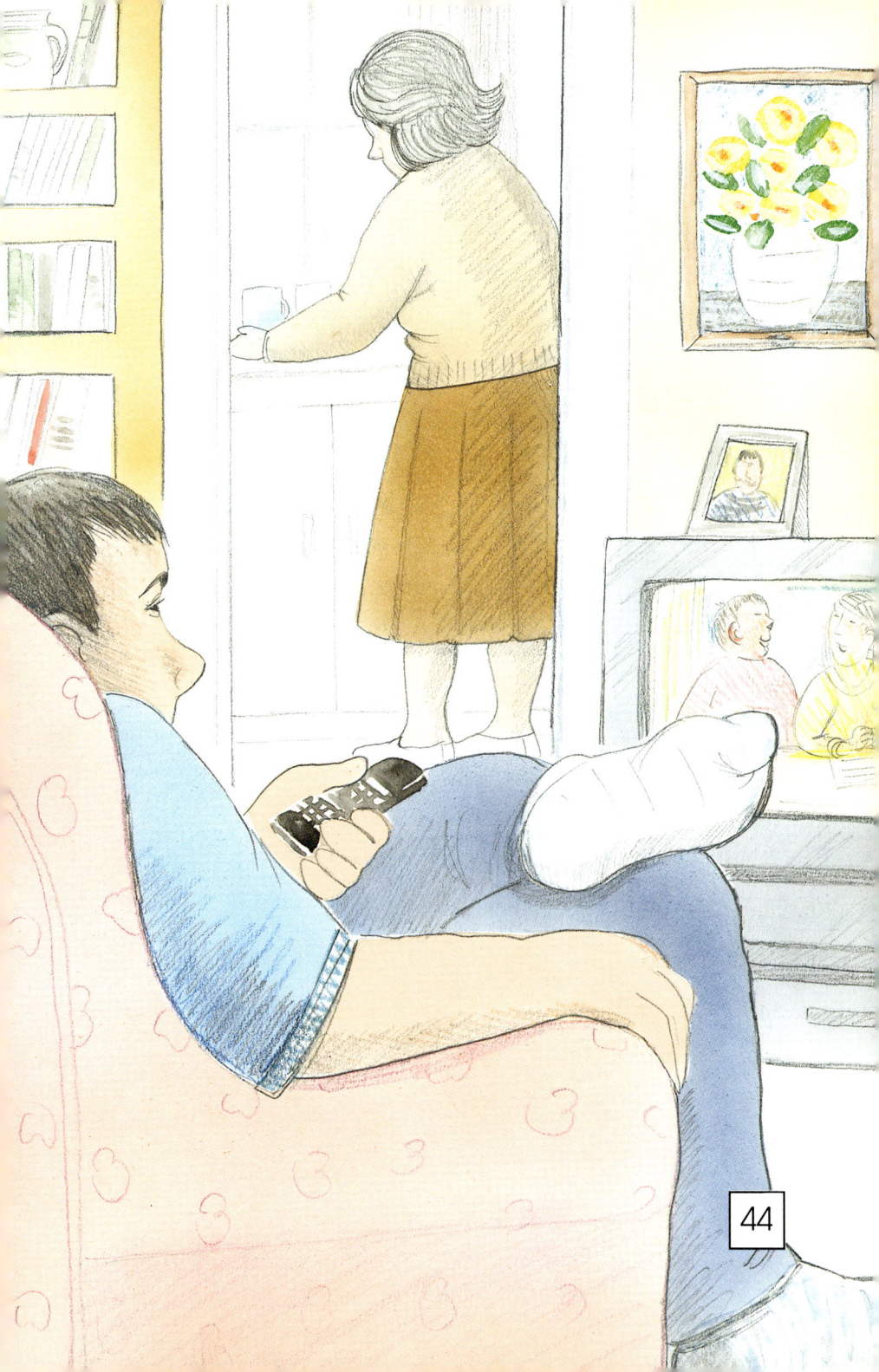

45

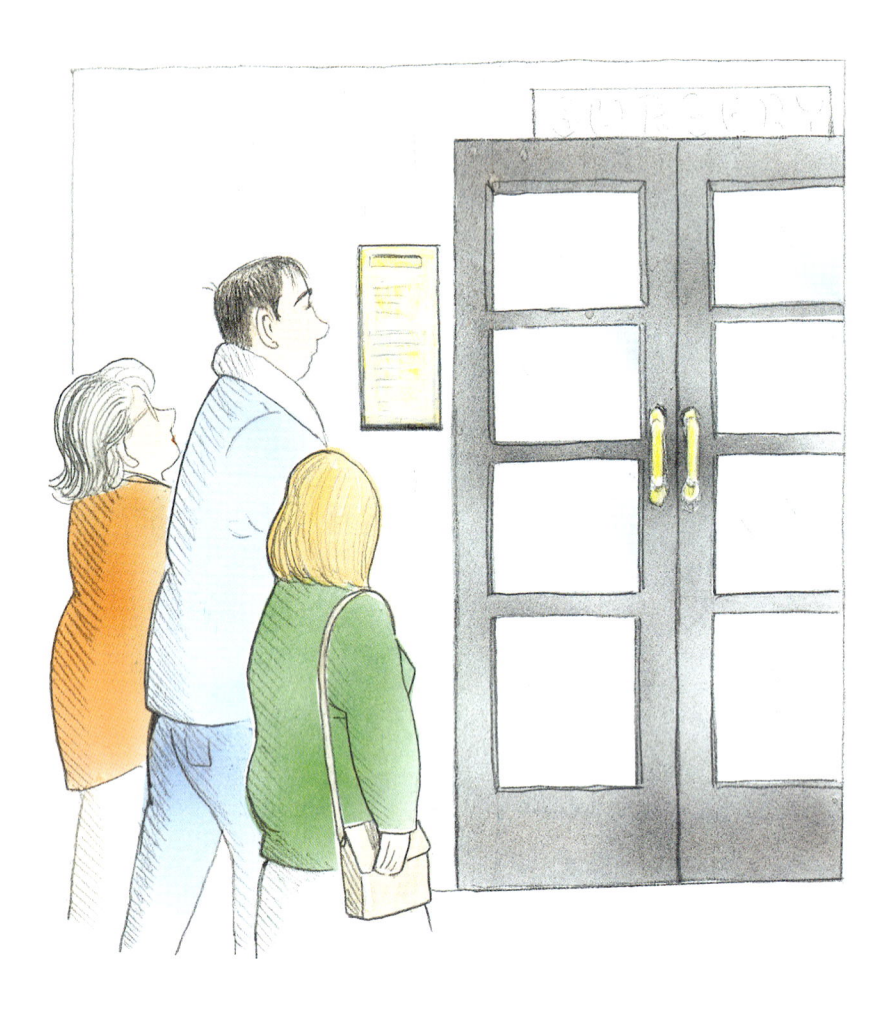

46

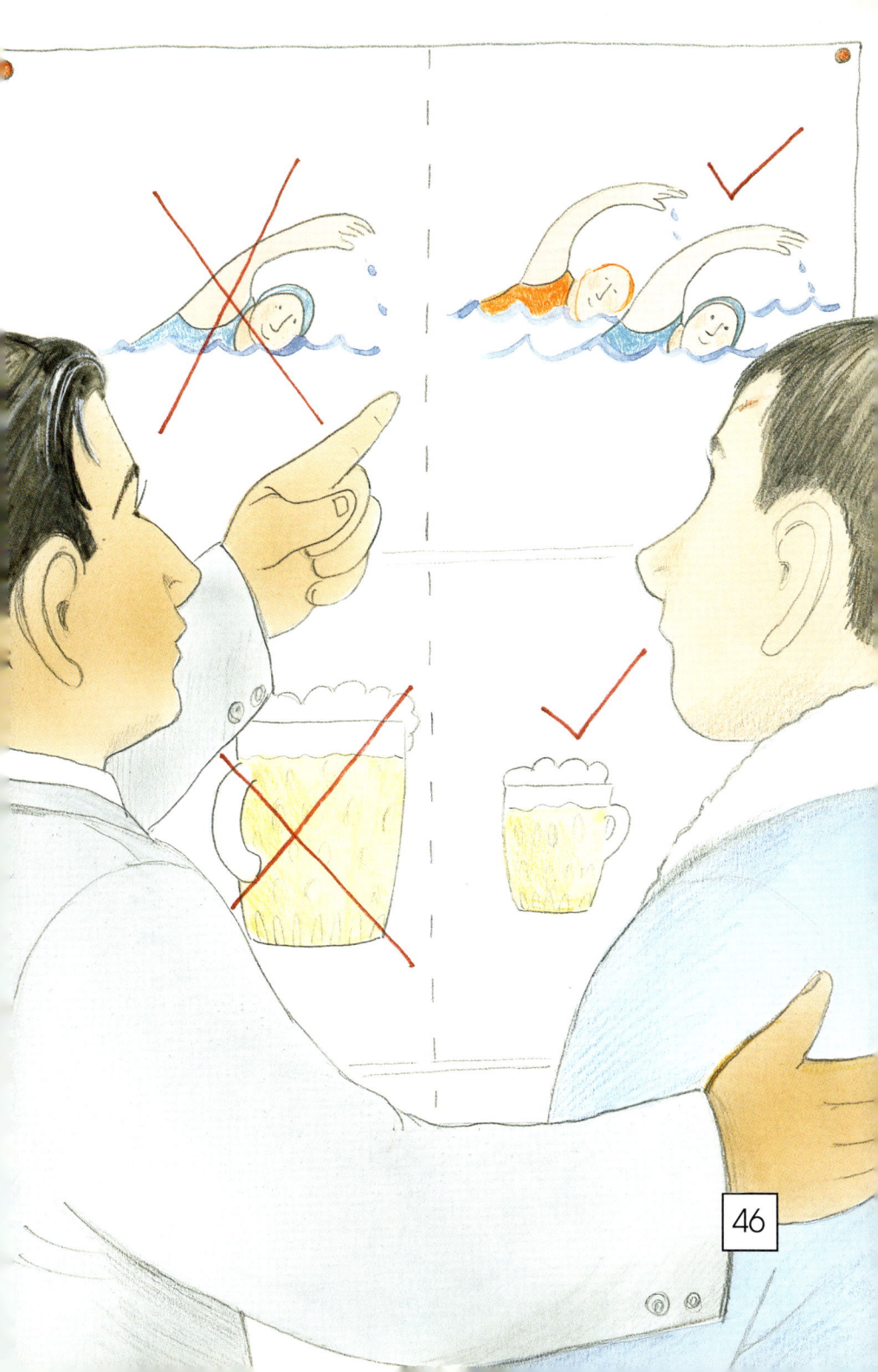

47

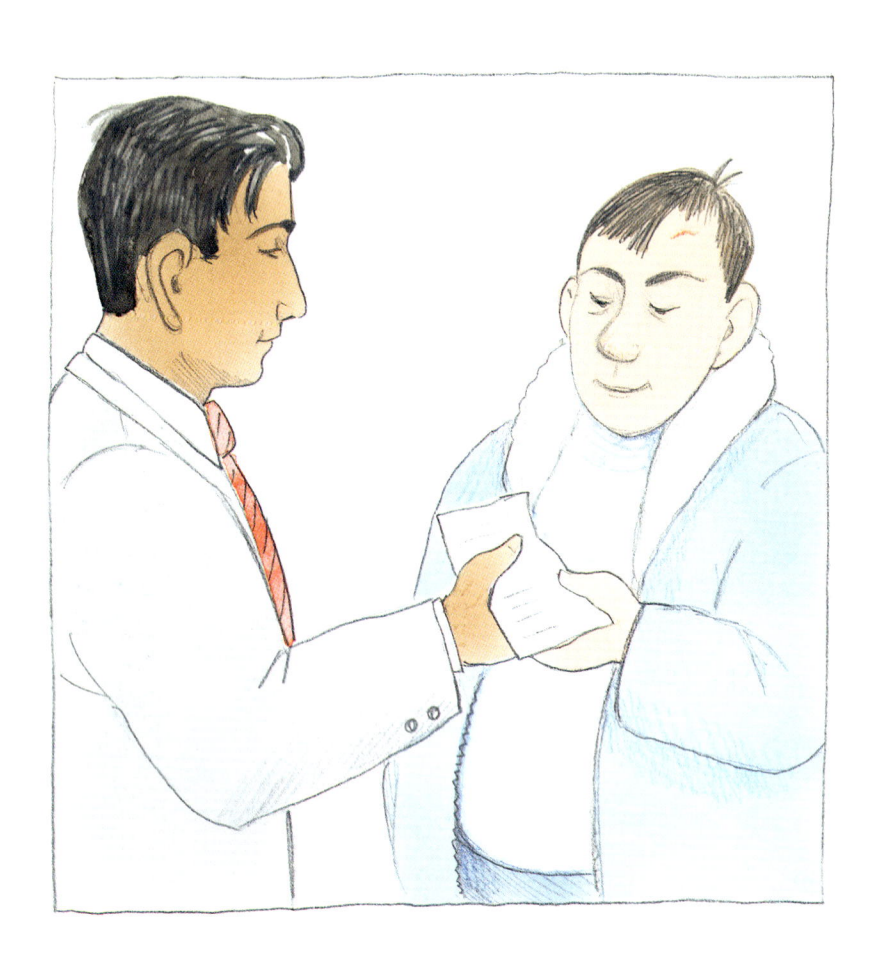

48

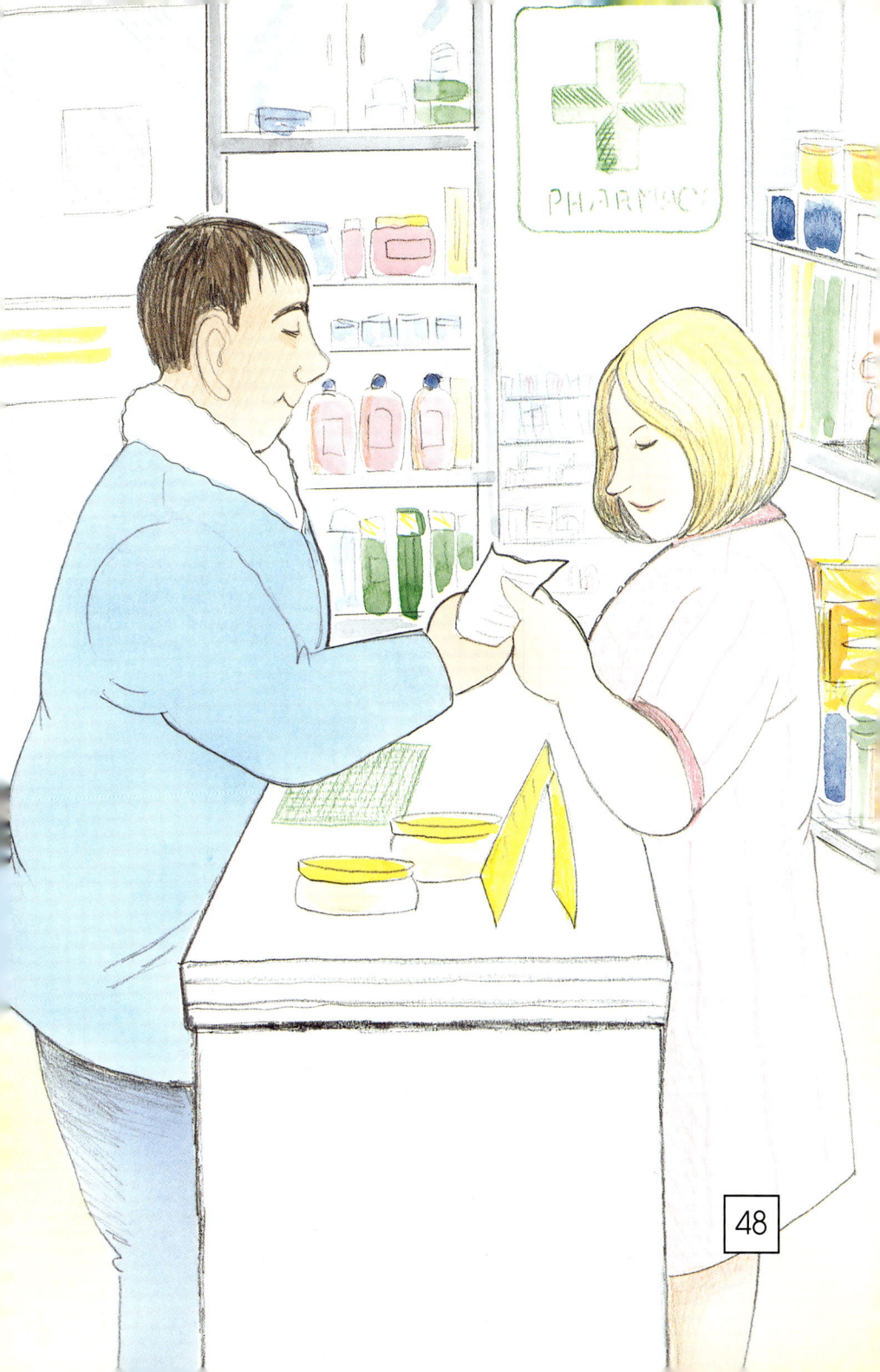

49

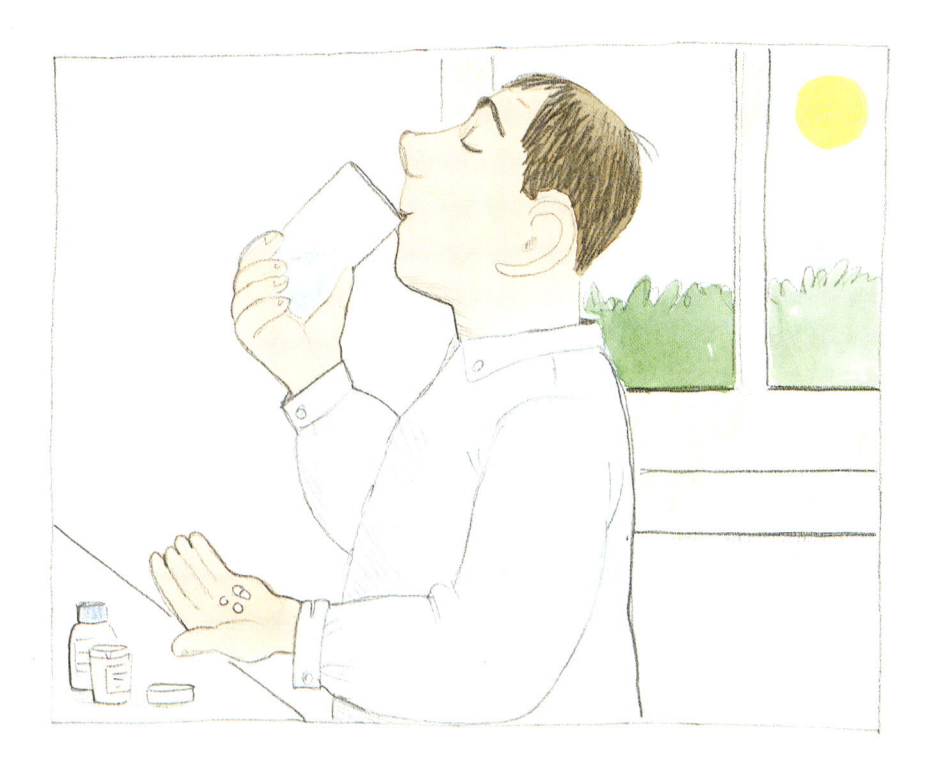

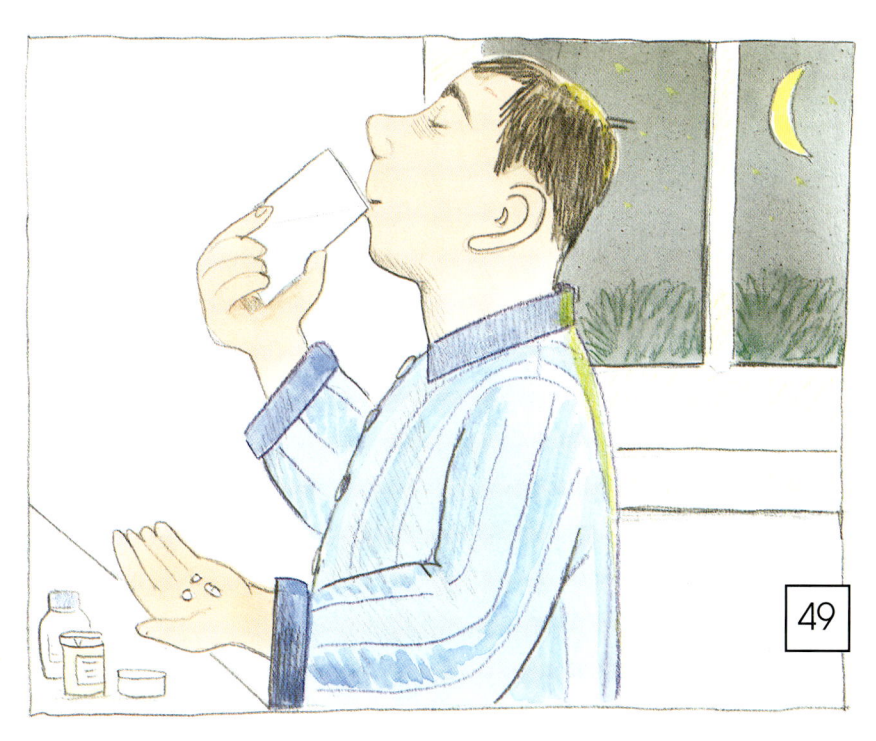

50

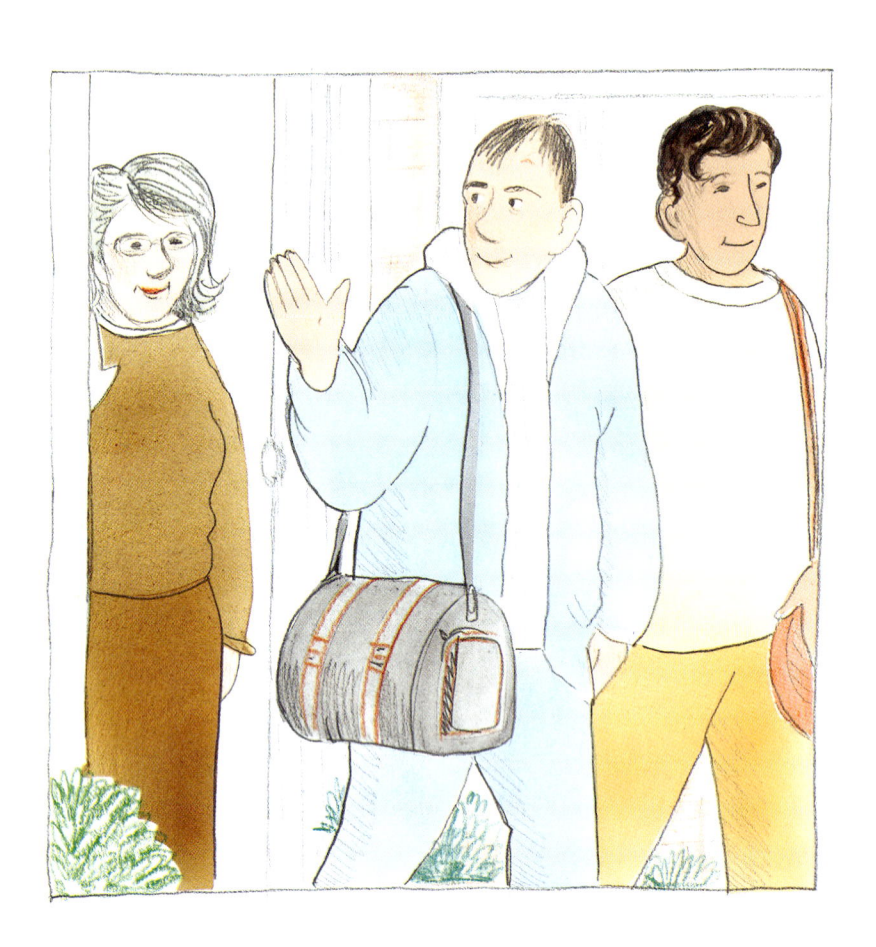

51

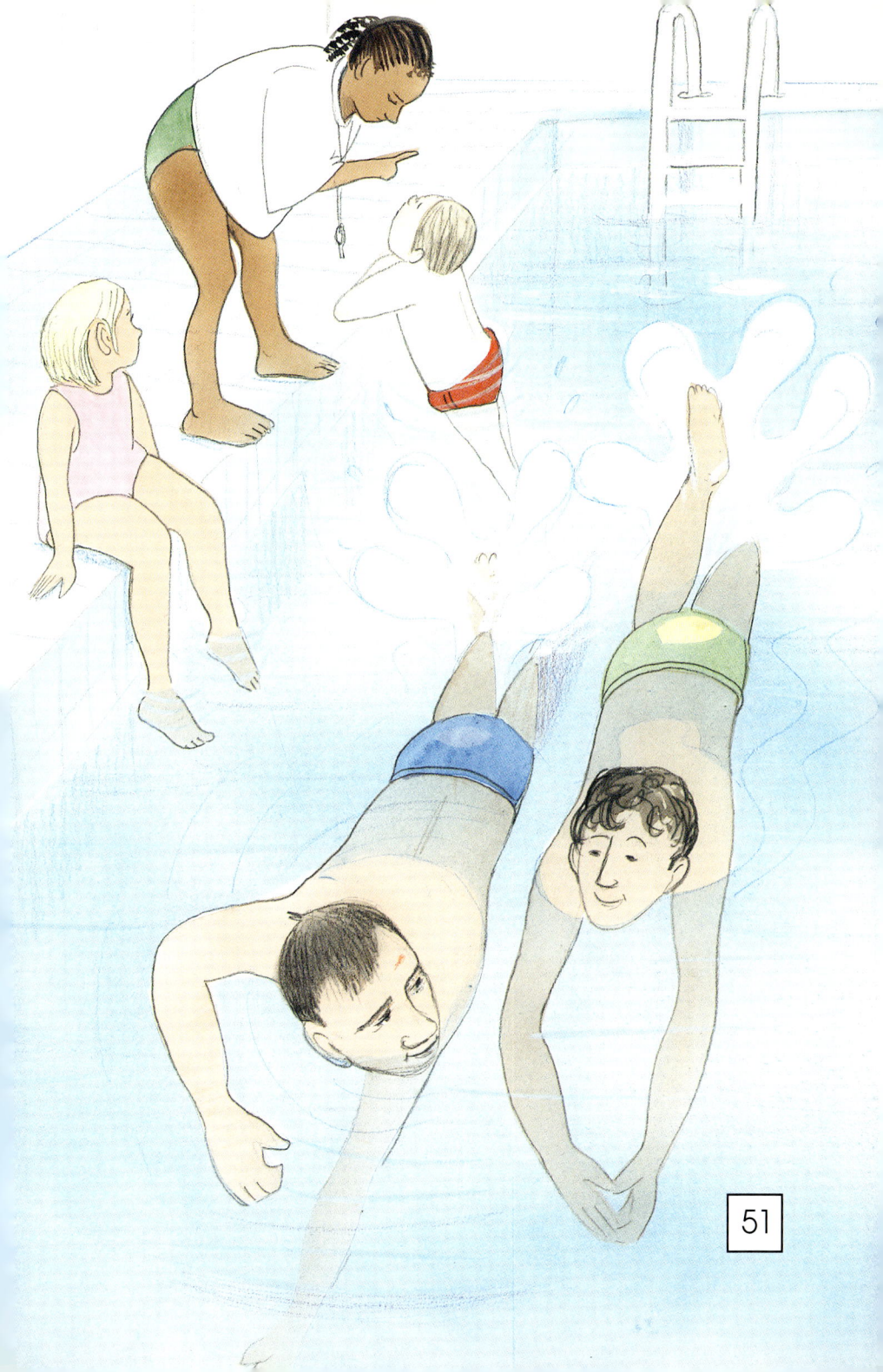

52

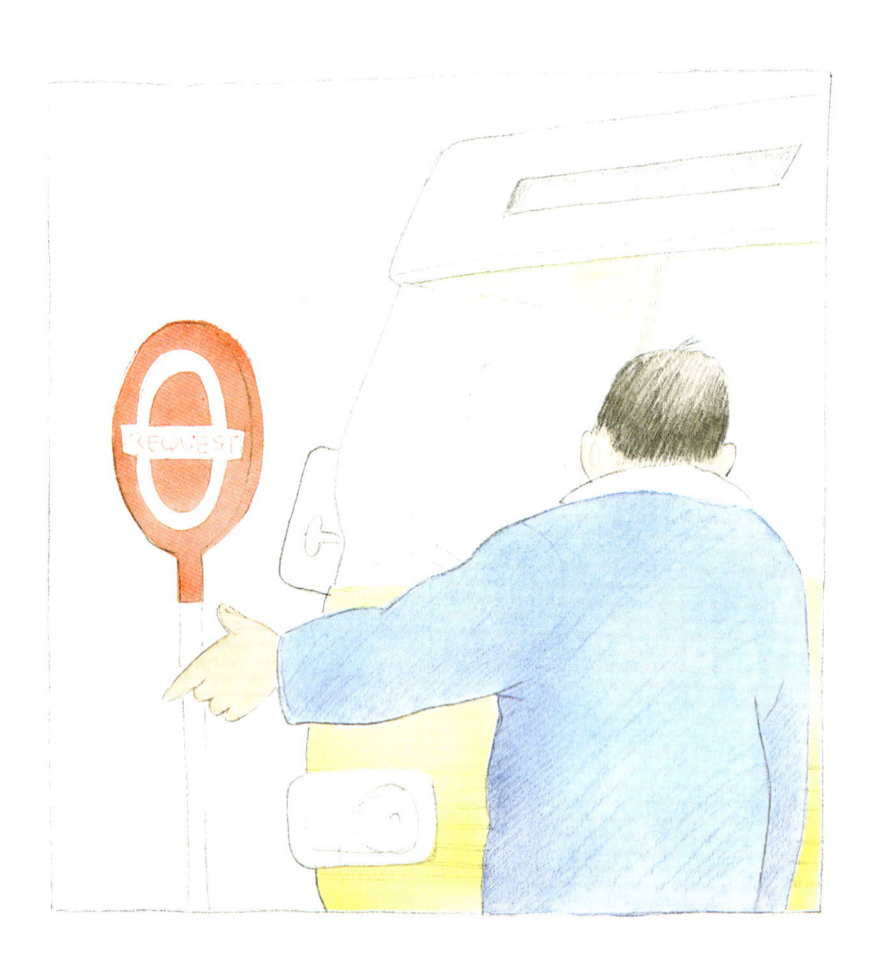

53

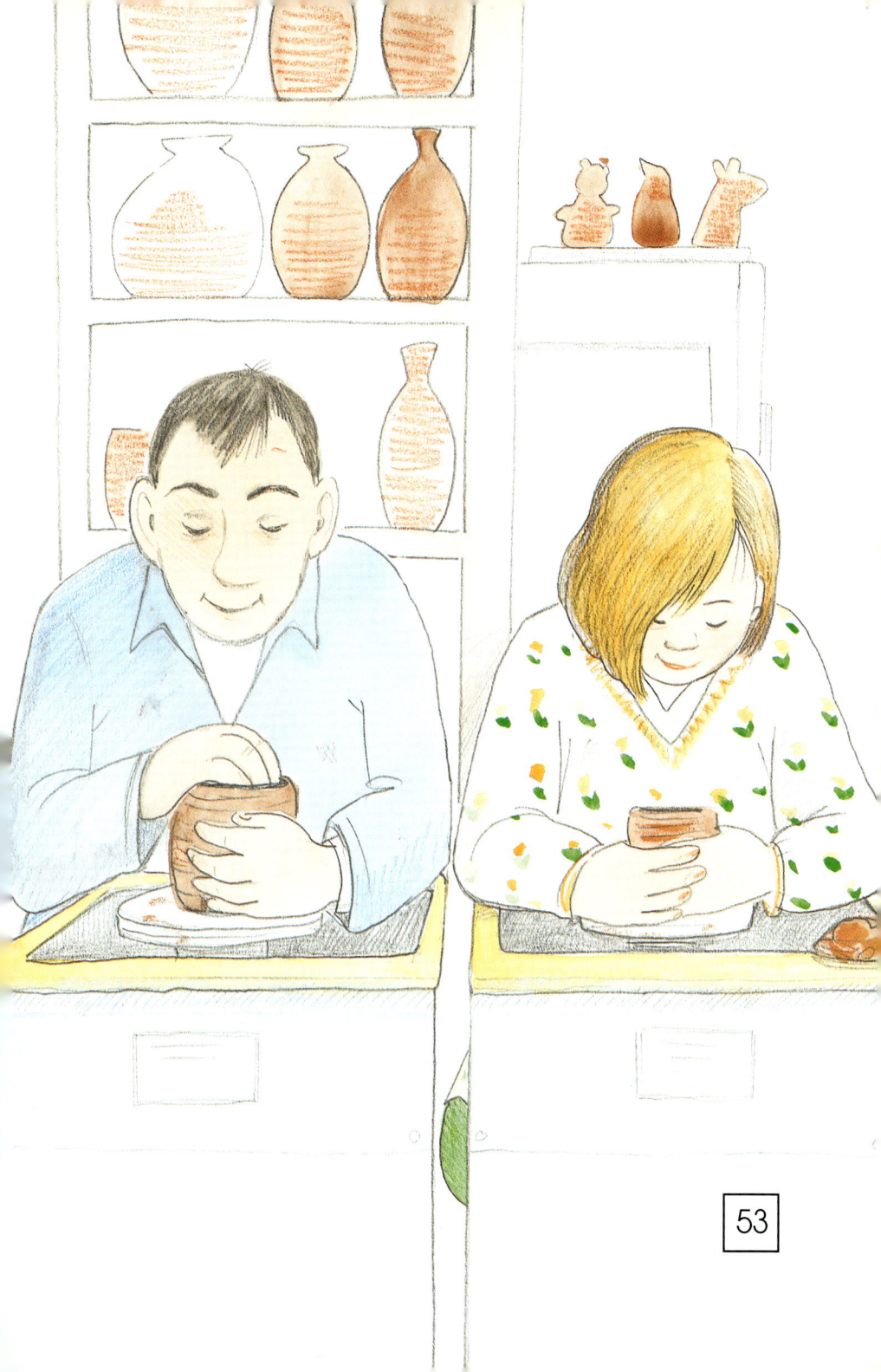

54

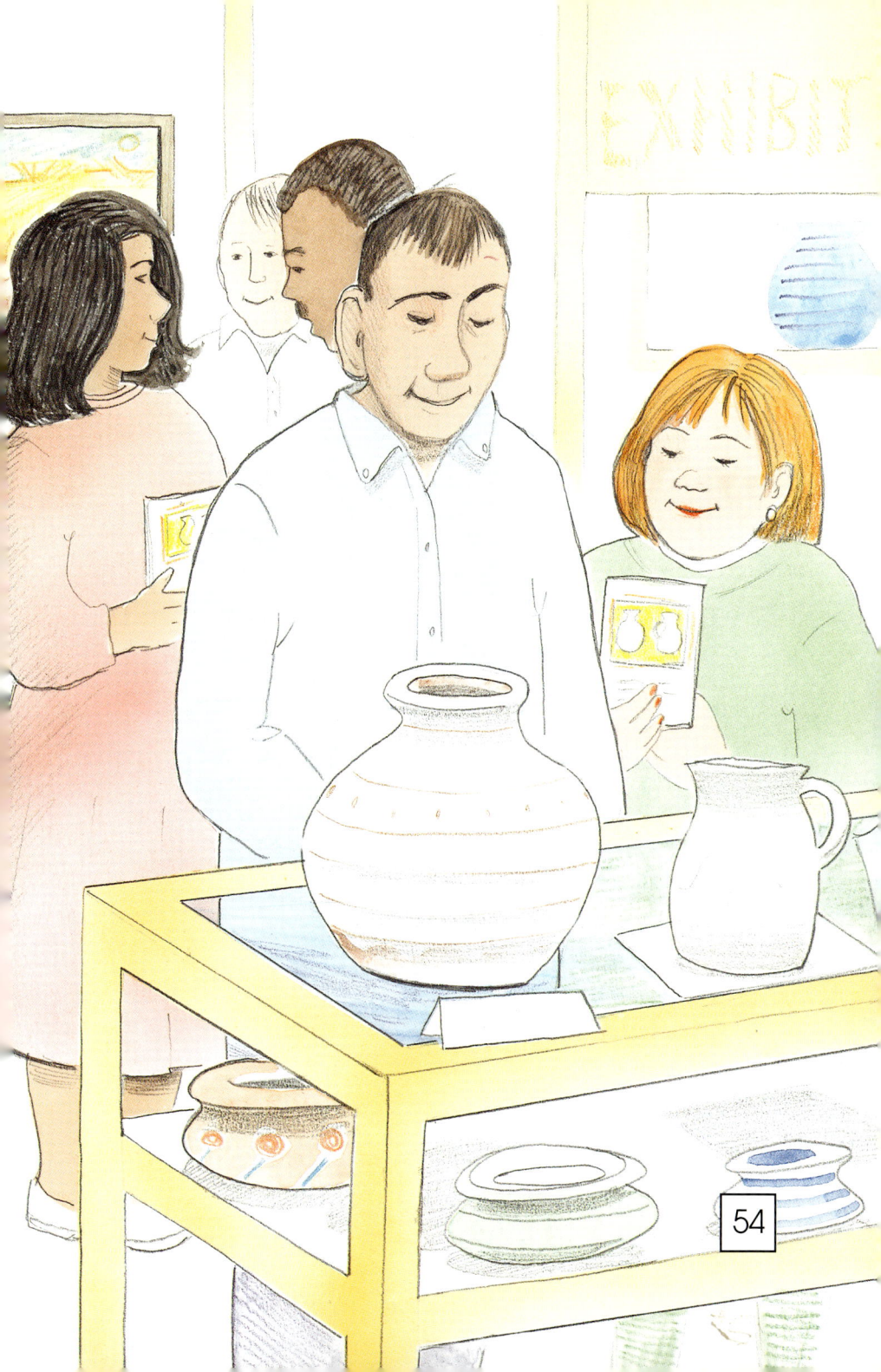

The following words are provided for readers or carers who want a ready-made story rather than to make up their own.

Picture numbers

1. Jack is waiting for the bus. The bus comes.
2. Jack gets on the bus. He enjoys looking out the window.
3. Jack gets off the bus at his stop.
4. Suddenly Jack's body goes stiff and starts shaking. He falls over. He is having a fit.
5. Jack is on the pavement, having a fit. His body is shaking. He does not know it is happening. Some people come to look at him. They are all worried. Some of them are scared. The bus driver rings for an ambulance on his mobile phone.
6. Jack's fit is over. He wakes up. His forehead is bleeding. He hurt his head on the pavement when he fell. He does not remember what happened.
7. The ambulance arrives.
8. The ambulance staff put a blanket around Jack. They help him get into the ambulance.
9. The ambulance takes Jack to the hospital Accident and Emergency Department.
10. A doctor in Accident and Emergency is cleaning the cut on Jack's head. A nurse rings up Jack's mother to tell her what happened.
11. The nurse tells Jack's mother that he had a fit. Jack's mother is worried.
12. Jack's mother comes to the hospital to see him. Jack has a plaster on the cut on his head.
13. Jack's mother helps him get into the car to go home.

14. At home, Jack's mother makes him a cup of tea. Jack feels fed-up about having a fit.
15. That evening, someone rings the doorbell.
16. Jack opens the door. His girlfriend, Sandy, and his other friend, Edward, are there. They ask Jack to go to the pub with them.
17. Jack's mother is worried. She does not want him to go out. He has had a fit already that day. She is afraid that he will have another fit. She tells him not to go. Jack decides to go out anyway.
18. Jack, Sandy and Edward go to the pub.
19. Jack drinks half a pint of beer. Edward drinks a pint. They have a good chat.
20. Jack says "Good night" to his friends.
21. Jack's mother asks him "What time do you call this then?!". She is worried that he has stayed out too late.
22. The next morning Jack and his mother have breakfast.
23. Jack waits for the bus to go to work.
24. Jack and Sandy are making pots.
25. Suddenly, Jack has another fit. He falls off his stool.
26. Sandy knows how to help Jack. She puts a soft coat under his head. When he stops shaking Sandy rolls him onto his side. This helps him to breathe.
27. Jack wakes up after the fit. Sandy comforts him.
28. Sandy helps Jack up. The other people are worried about him.
29. Sandy helps Jack go home.
30. Jack's mother rings the doctor to tell him about Jack's fits.

31. Jack, his mother and Sandy all go to see the doctor.
32. The doctor says "Hello" to Jack.
33. Sandy tells the doctor about Jack's fit at work.
34. Jack shows the doctor the tablets he takes.
35. The doctor explains to Jack about epilepsy. They look at a picture book.
36. The doctor says that Jack must have some tests. The doctor shows him pictures of the tests.
37. Jack and his mother go to the hospital.
38. At the hospital, Jack has a test called an '**EEG**' (electroencephalogram). It takes about an hour. Jack lies down on a table. The EEG lady sticks wires on his head. It does not hurt at all. The wires go into a big machine. The machine draws squiggly lines on a long paper. Later the doctor looks at the lines. He can see if Jack has epilepsy.
39. Then Jack goes to have an MRI brain scan. It's like a very big camera. It will take a picture of Jack's brain. The **radiographer** (staff) tells Jack what will happen.
40. Jack lies down inside the big machine. He must stay still or the picture will come out blurry. The machine fits snugly around him. It is very noisy. It does not hurt. The test takes half an hour. Jack can see the radiographer all the time. She stays near the machine to look after him.
41. Next, Jack goes to the blood test clinic.
42. The nurse takes some of Jack's blood to test it. The needle pricks his arm. The blood goes into a bottle.
43. Jack and his mother leave the hospital. They are glad that the tests are finished.
44. That evening Jack relaxes at home as usual.
45. Two weeks later Jack goes back to see the doctor. His mother and Sandy go with him.

46. The doctor tells Jack that the tests show that Jack has epilepsy. The doctor shows Jack pictures of things he can and can't do to stay safe and well. He should not swim by himself. He *can* go swimming if there is someone with him. Jack should not drink a whole pint of lager. He can drink *one half* pint in an evening.

47. The doctor gives Jack a prescription. He has written on the prescription what tablets Jack should take.

48. Jack goes to the chemist and gives in the prescription.

49. Every day Jack takes two tablets and one capsule in the morning when he gets up. He takes two tablets and one capsule before he goes to bed at night.

50. One day Jack decides to go swimming. He asks his friend to go with him.

51. Jack and his friend enjoy swimming together.

52. During the week Jack catches the bus to work. He is not afraid to travel on the bus.

53. Jack and Sandy make beautiful pottery.

54. There is a pottery exhibition. Lots of people come to look at the pots. Jack and Sandy are proud to show off their work.

What is epilepsy?

Jack has epilepsy. People with epilepsy are people who sometimes have a **fit**. Fits are also called **seizures**, **turns**, **blackouts** or **attacks**. Doctors prefer to call them seizures. A fit happens when someone's brain suddenly stops working properly for a short time. If somebody has just one fit in their whole life, they do not have epilepsy.

What is a fit?

In the story Jack has two fits. Different people have different kinds of fits. Some people fall over, then their body starts to jerk. They are not awake. They may wet themselves. They may dirty themselves. That is the kind of fit Jack has. Other people may get shakes in just one arm or leg. Some people know when they are going to have a fit. They may get a funny feeling in their tummy or a funny taste. They call this a warning, or **aura**. Some people get no warning. Some people may undress themselves in the street or do something else that is unusual for them. Some people are awake when they have a fit. Other people do not even know they have had a fit until someone else tells them. They were not awake. They do not remember having a fit. A few people have more than one kind of fit.

What causes a fit?

All epileptic fits start off in the brain. The brain controls our movements. The brain controls whether we are asleep or awake. It sorts out what we see, hear or smell. All our thoughts come from our brains. The brain is made of smaller parts called cells. The different parts of the brain send electrical messages to one another. Sometimes far too many messages are sent out all at once. The brain cannot sort out so many messages. It suddenly stops working properly for a few seconds. When that happens in someone's brain the person has an epileptic fit. After a few seconds the brain goes back to its usual way of working.

An epileptic fit is not the same as being angry or sad. It is not the same as not understanding. People do not have epileptic fits on purpose. People with epilepsy cannot usually control when they have fits.

Why do some people have epilepsy?

Doctors do not always know exactly what causes a person's epilepsy. They do know it starts in the person's brain. It can be caused by a scar or by other damage in their brain.

Epilepsy is more common in people with learning disabilities. But most people with epilepsy do not have learning disabilities. Most people with learning disabilities do not have epilepsy.

People with epilepsy can

- Work.
- Do sports.
- Go swimming.
- Party.
- Use computers.
- Cook.
- Travel.

Sometimes they may need to take extra care so they don't have an accident. See pictures later in this book.

What to do if someone has a fit (1)

Sandy knows what to do when Jack has a fit. If you see someone have a fit what should you do? You have to decide who is the best person to help. Sometimes a supporter or a first-aider may be there. If you have to manage on your own, this is what to do:

- Do not leave the person alone. **Try not to feel frightened**. Once an epileptic fit has started, nobody can stop it. It will stop on its own.
- Keep the person safe until the fit stops.

During the fit

- Stop other people from crowding round.
- Ask for help if you need it.
- Put something soft under the person's head (like a jacket or cardigan) to stop them hurting themselves.
- Do **not** try to move the person unless you really have to. If they are in a very dangerous place, like the middle of the road, ask someone else to help you. They can keep the traffic away or help you move the person who is having a fit.
- Do **not** put anything in the person's mouth. There is no danger of them swallowing their tongue and you could easily break their teeth by mistake.

Once the jerking has stopped

- Roll the person on their side in the recovery position.
- If the person is not breathing properly, check that nothing is blocking their throat like false teeth or food.
- Do not make a big fuss if the person has wet themselves.
- Stay talking to them until they feel better.

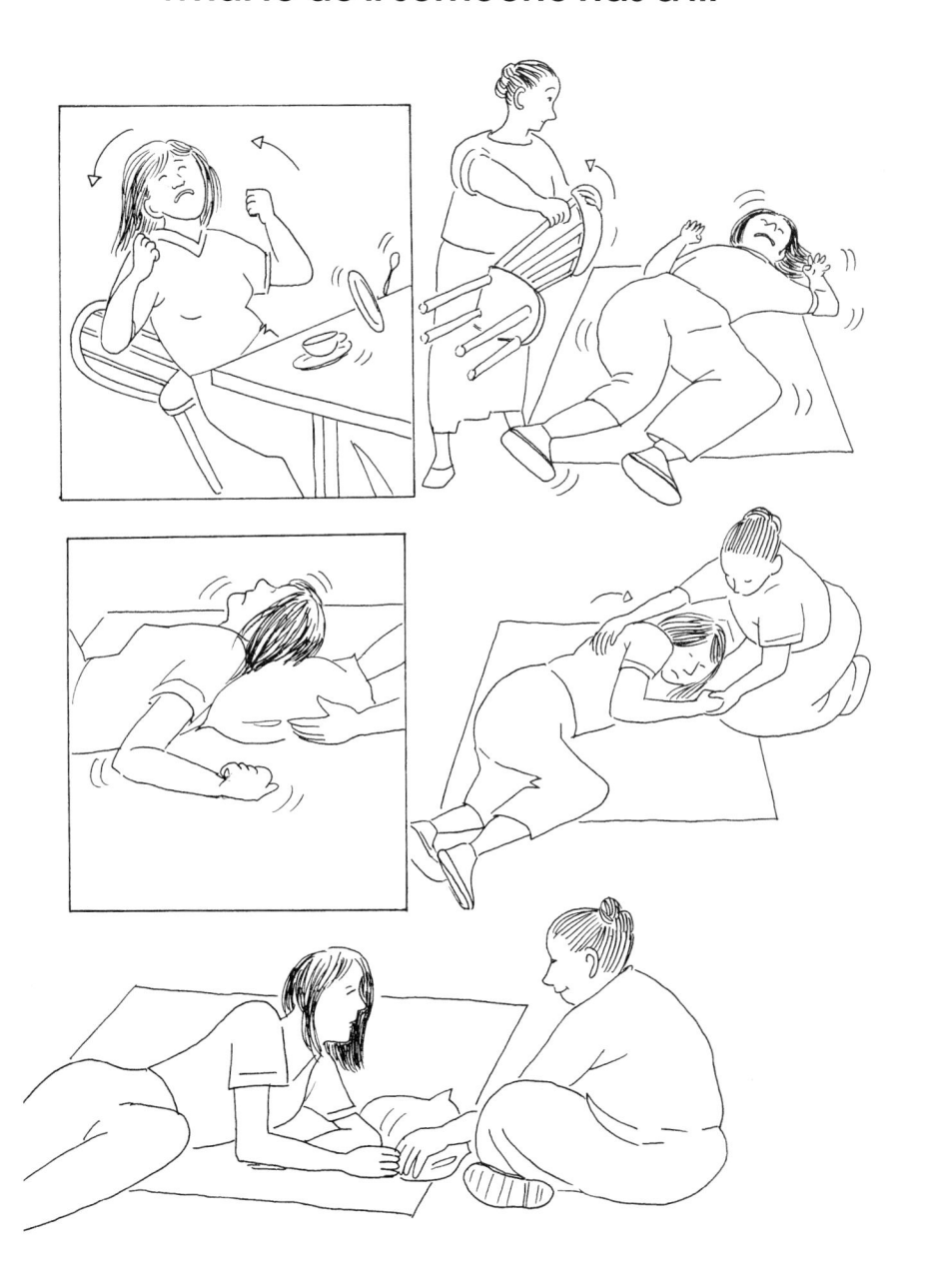

What to do if someone has a fit

What to do if someone has a fit (2)

Other sorts of fits

For example, if the person seems muddled:

- Gently guide them away from doing anything dangerous like wandering in the road.
- Keep other people from crowding round.
- Speak gently and calmly to the person. This will help them sort out what is happening.
- Remember that the person may be muddled for some time after the fit. They may seem angry or moody.
- Stay with the person until they are back to their usual self.

Ask someone to call an ambulance if:

- The person has hurt themselves badly in a fit.
- The person has trouble breathing after a fit.
- The person has another fit straight after.
- The fit goes on longer than that person's fits usually do.
- You don't know how long that person's fits usually go on for, and this fit has gone on for more than five minutes

Taking tablets, capsules or medicines

The doctor writes down your medicine, tablets or capsules on a piece of paper called a prescription. You take the prescription to the chemist who gives you the medicine the doctor has written down.
Anti-epileptic drugs or **anticonvulsant drugs** are tablets or medicine that the doctor prescribes for epilepsy. You take

anti-epileptic drugs to *prevent* fits. The anti-epileptic drugs can not stop a fit once it has started. If you take anti-epileptic drugs regularly they will stop you from having more fits. It is very important to take anti-epileptic drugs exactly as your doctor tells you to. It is dangerous to stop taking them suddenly without asking your doctor. If you think the drugs are not working or they are making you feel ill, tell your doctor.

The doctor will tell you:

- What the tablets are for.
- The time of day to take them.
- How to take them; how long to go on taking them.
- What to do if you miss a dose.
- Whether you can drink alcohol while you are taking the tablets.
- Whether you can use machinery when you are taking the tablets.
- What side-effects the tablets may have.
- Who to ask if you are worried.

Side-effects

The doctor prescribes tablets or medicine to help you. Sometimes the tablets or medicine also have bad effects. These are called side-effects. Side-effects are when the tablets or medicine you take make you feel ill. Some side-effects are: feeling sleepy, feeling sick or getting a rash. If you get side-effects, tell your doctor. You may need different tablets or medicine.

You can photocopy these drawings and insert your own text to fit the advice you are giving. See the examples below.

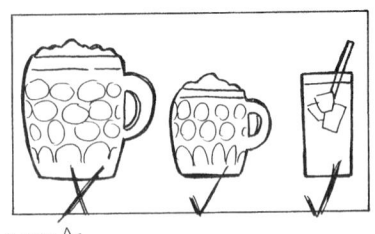

EMMA
IT'S OK TO DRINK ONE SMALL BEER, MORE THAN THAT COULD MAKE YOUR FITS WORSE

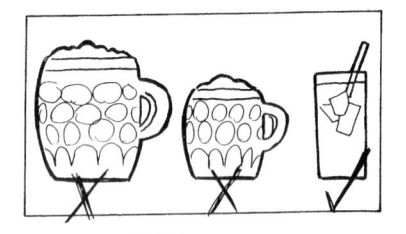

GEORGE
PLEASE DO NOT DRINK ANY BEER. DRINK FRUIT JUICE OR ANOTHER, NON-ALCOHOLIC DRINK

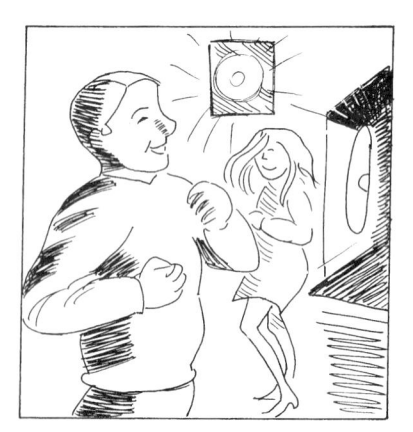

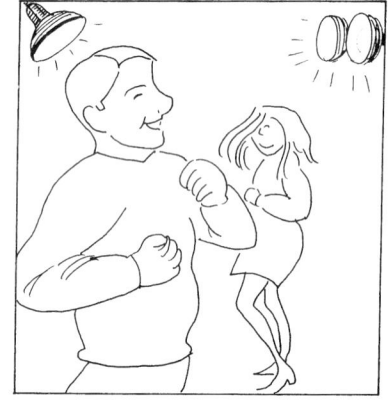

JACK IT'S OK FOR YOU TO GO TO THE DISCO AND DANCE. SOME PEOPLE WITH EPILEPSY HAVE MORE FITS WITH DISCO LIGHTS — YOU DON'T HAVE THAT SORT OF EPILEPSY. HAVE FUN AT THE DISCO!

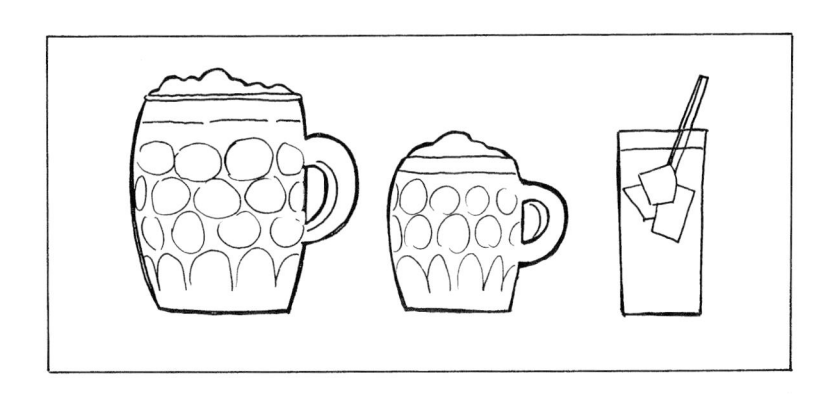

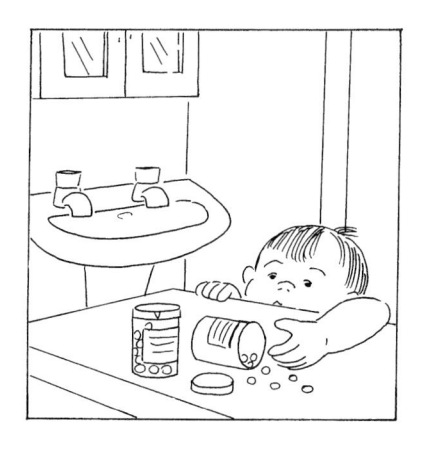

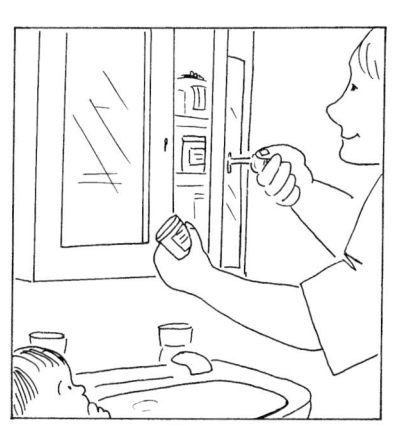

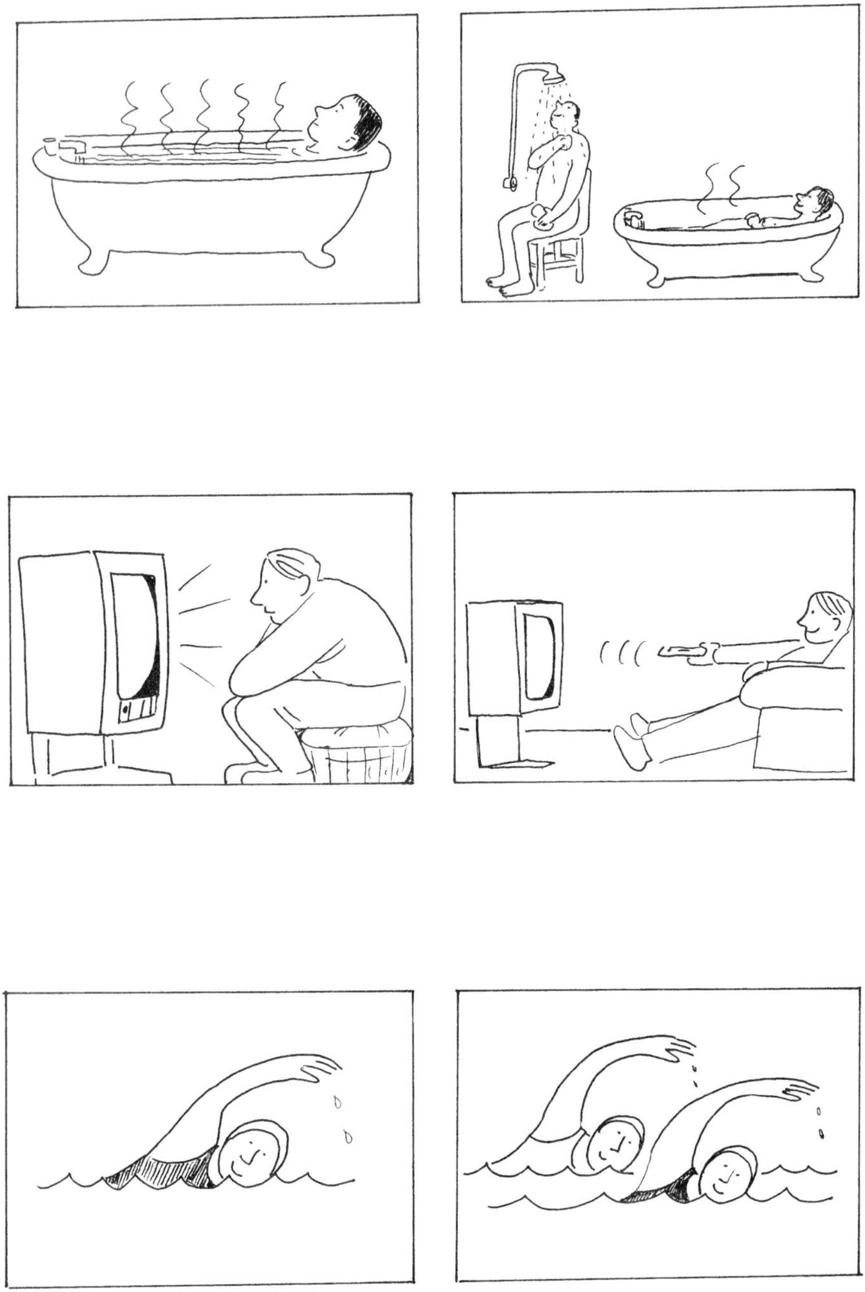

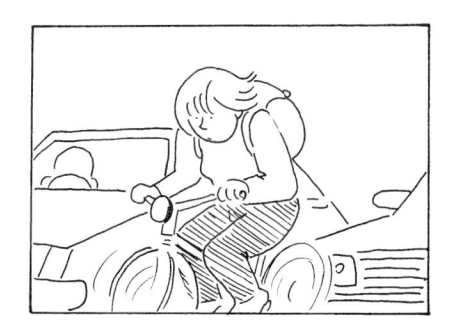

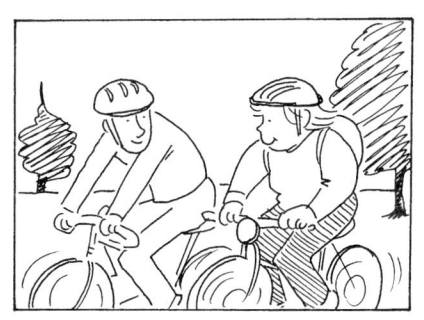

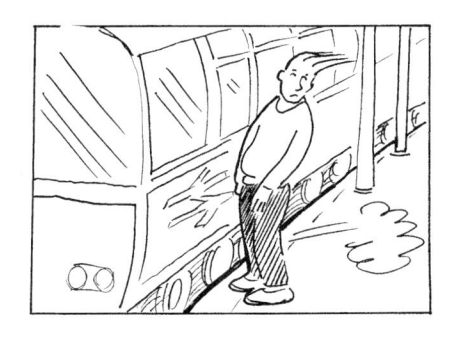

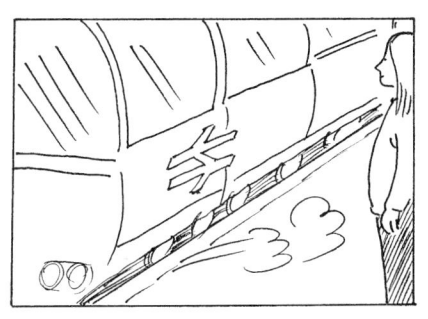

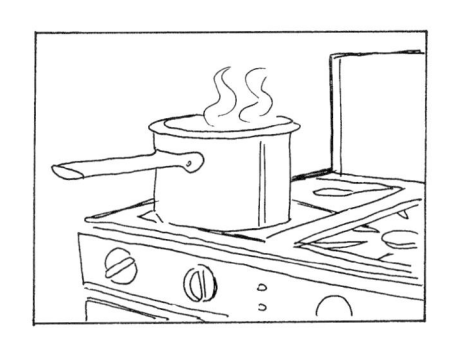

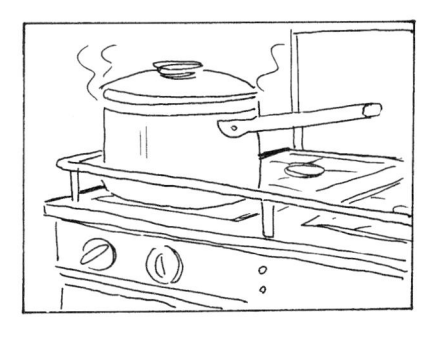

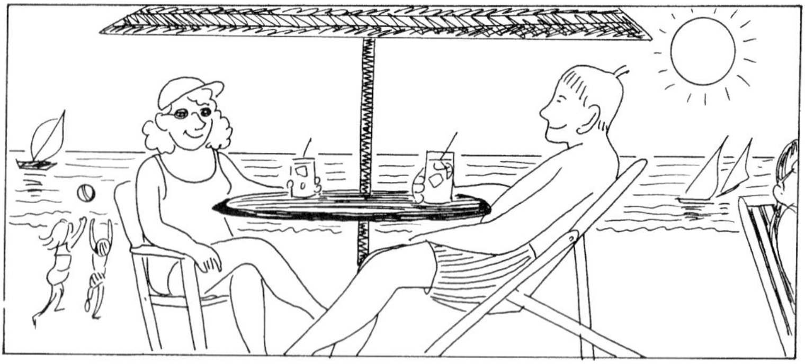

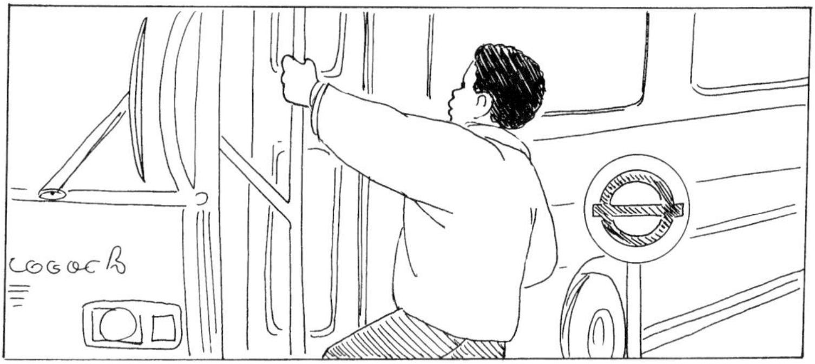

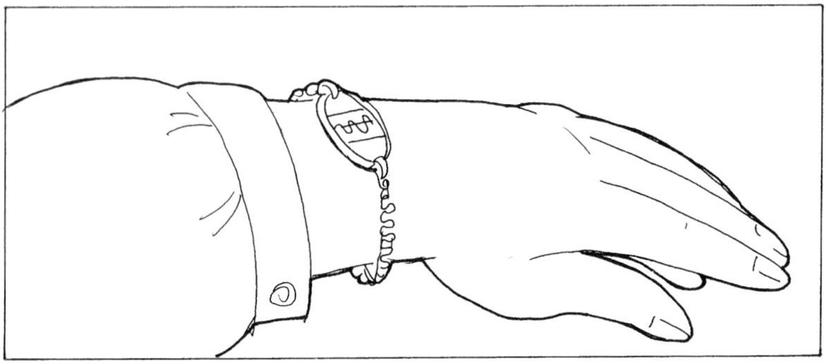

The Clinic

You can photocopy these drawings and insert your own text to fit the advice you are giving.

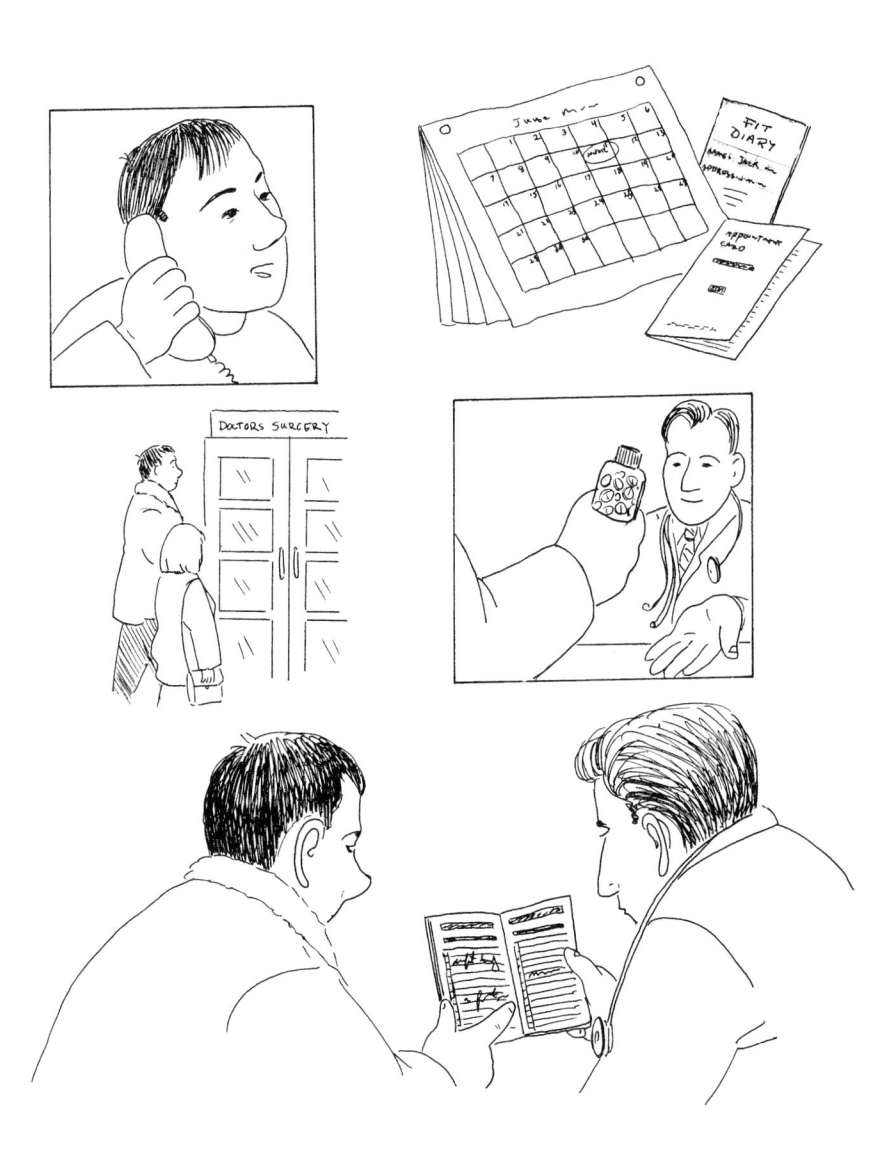

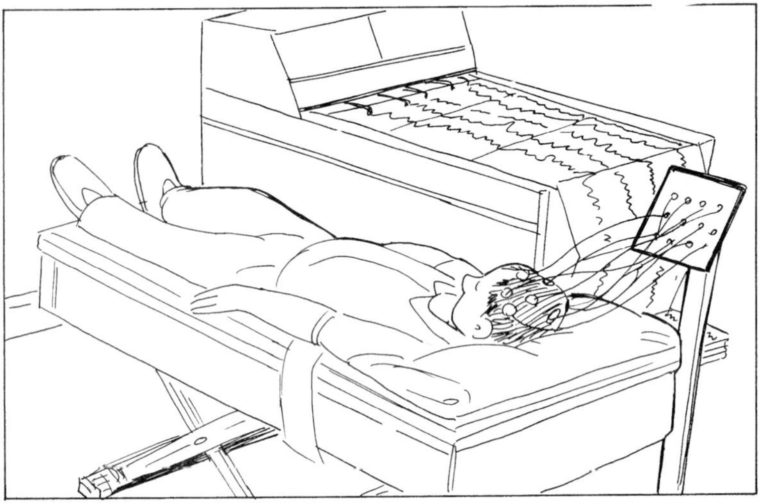

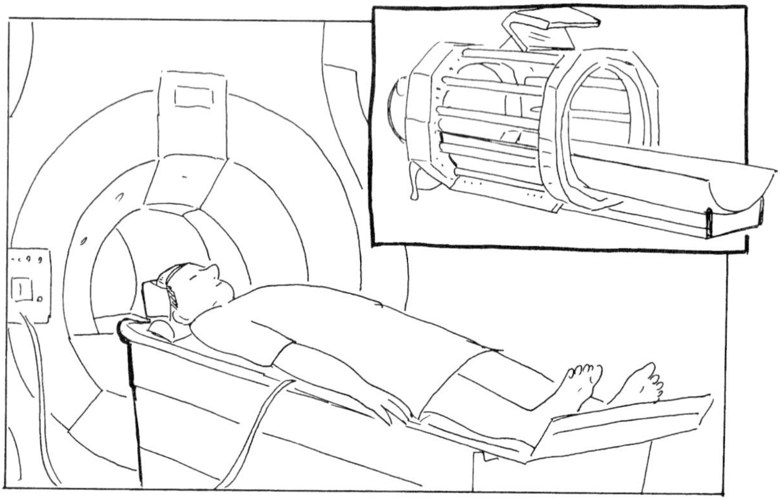

Your prescription

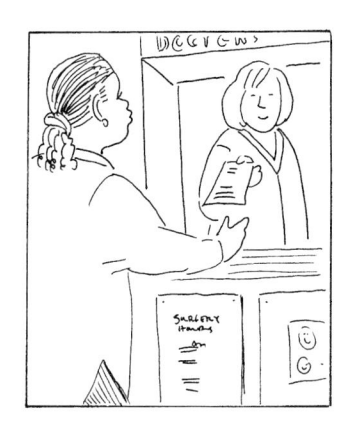

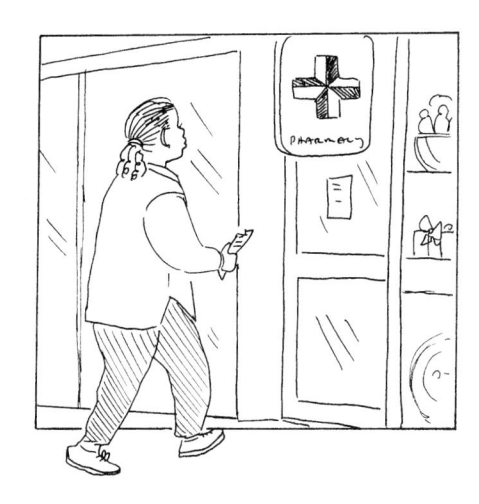

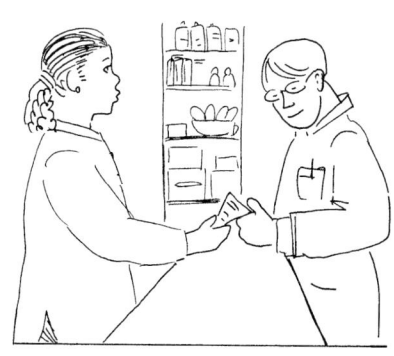

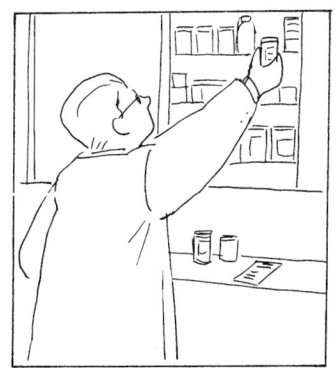

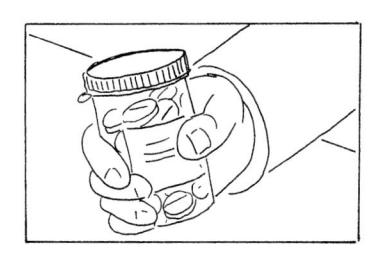

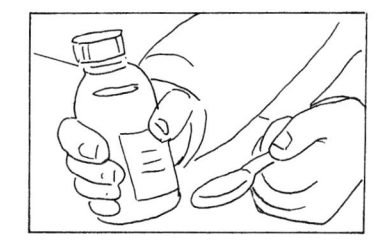

Useful resources

Services

Epilepsy Clinics Sometimes these are run by Neurology Departments, sometimes by Learning Disability Services.

Community Teams for People with Learning Disabilities (CTPLDs) These are specialist multi-disciplinary health teams that support adults with learning disabilities and their families by assessment of their health needs and a range of clinical interventions.

Who to contact for help and advice

British Epilepsy Association　　　　　　0113 210 8800
National Information Centre　　　　　　(0808 8005050
New Anstey House　　　　　　　freephone helpline)
Gateway Drive　　　　Website: www.epilepsy.org.uk
Yeadon
Leeds LS3 1BE

Epilepsy Association of Scotland　　　　0141 427 4911
48 Govan Road
Glasgow
G51 1JL

Medic Alert　　　　　　　　　　　　0171 833 3034
1 Bridge Wharf
156 Caledonian Road
London
N1 9UU

For identity bracelets and necklaces.

Mersey Region Epilepsy Association　　0151 298 2666
Glaxo Neurological Centre
Norton Street
Liverpool L3 8LR

The National Society for Epilepsy 01494 601400
Chalfont St Peter (helpline)
Gerrards Cross
Buckinghamshire
SK9 0RJ

Written material

Department of Health (1998) *Signposts for Success in Commissioning and Providing Health Services for People with Learning Disabilities*. Contains examples of, and advice on, good practice.

Epilepsy: what is epilepsy; what causes it; *What to Do When Someone has a Fit* by Roslyn Band. Paperback, £8.00. From The Elfrida Society, 34 Islington Park Street, London N1 1PX.

First Aid Manual. Dr Michael Webb, Sir Michael Bond & Sir Peter Beale. Published by Dorling Kindersley Ltd at £10.99. ISBN: 0-7513-0707-6 (paperback).

Video material

Epilepsy and You by Audrey Paul. A programme to help people with learning disabilities understand and manage their epilepsy. Format: video (11 minutes) and guidance booklet (16 pp). £35 plus VAT (total £41.12) From: Pavilion Publishing, 8 St George's Place, FREEPOST BR 458, Brighton, East Sussex BN1 4ZZ.

Website

The website includes standard letters, charts and black and white illustrations, including those provided in this book for use in an epilepsy clinic. This is also available at: *www.rcpsych.ac.uk*

Books Beyond Words

A range of other titles is available in this series.

Three books cover access to criminal justice as a victim (witness) or as a defendant: **Going to Court**, **You're Under Arrest** and **You're on Trial**.

Using health services, including the GP, is explained in **Going to the Doctor**, **Going to Out-Patients** and **Going into Hospital**.

Feeling Blue is aimed at helping people to understand depression.

Michelle Finds a Voice explains methods of augmentative communication.

The difficult subject of sexual abuse is covered in **Bob Tells All**, **Jenny Speaks Out**, and **I Can Get Through It**. Counselling and psychotherapy after sexual abuse are explained in the third title.

Peter's New Home and **A New Home in the Community** help explain about moving home.

Forming new relationships is the subject of **Making Friends** and **Hug Me Touch Me**. The ups and downs of a romantic relationship are traced in **Falling in Love**.

When Dad Died and **When Mum Died** help people to understand bereavement.

The books are priced at £10 each. To order copies, or a leaflet giving more information about these books, please contact: Book Sales, Royal College of Psychiatrists, 17 Belgrave Square, London SW1X 8PG. Credit card orders can be taken by telephone (+44 (0)207 235 2351, ext. 146).